THE ULTIMATE DIABETIC COOKBOOK FOR BEGINNERS

Step-By-Step Guide To 2000 Delicious Days Of Super Easy And Nutritious Diabetic Diet Recipes With A Complete Meal Plan For Type 1 & 2 Diabetes / Suitable For Newly Diagnosed And Prediabetic

Nathan Wendy

Table of Contents

COPYRIGHT © 2023

the prior written permission of the publisher, except in the case of brief quotations embodied in critical reviews and certain other noncommercial uses permitted by copyright law.

CHAPTER ONE

Understanding Diabetes and Nutrition

Diabetes is a chronic condition characterized by elevated levels of glucose (sugar) in the blood. Proper nutrition plays a crucial role in managing diabetes and preventing complications. This comprehensive guide aims to delve into various aspects of diabetes and nutrition, providing detailed insights into types of diabetes, blood sugar regulation, the importance of nutrition, and crafting a diabetic-friendly diet.

Introduction to Diabetes

Diabetes is a metabolic disorder that affects how your body uses blood sugar (glucose). Glucose is essential for providing energy to cells, and insulin, a hormone produced by the pancreas, helps regulate glucose levels in the blood. However, in individuals with diabetes, the body either does not produce enough insulin or cannot effectively use the insulin it produces.

Types of Diabetes

There are several types of diabetes, including:

1. **Type 1 Diabetes**: This type occurs when the immune system attacks and destroys the insulin-producing cells in the pancreas. As a result, the body produces little to no insulin. Type 1 diabetes is typically diagnosed in children and young adults, although it can develop at any age.

2. **Type 2 Diabetes**: In type 2 diabetes, the body becomes resistant to insulin or does not produce enough insulin to maintain normal glucose levels. This form of diabetes is more common and often develops in adults, although it is increasingly diagnosed in children and adolescents due to rising obesity rates and sedentary lifestyles.

3. **Gestational Diabetes**: This type of diabetes occurs during pregnancy when the body cannot produce enough insulin to meet the increased demands. Gestational diabetes usually

resolves after childbirth, but women who develop it are at higher risk of developing type 2 diabetes later in life.

4. **Prediabetes**: Prediabetes is a condition in which blood sugar levels are higher than normal but not yet high enough to be diagnosed as type 2 diabetes. Without intervention, prediabetes often progresses to type 2 diabetes.

Blood Sugar Regulation

In a healthy individual, blood sugar levels are tightly regulated to ensure they remain within a narrow range. When you eat carbohydrates, they are broken down into glucose, which enters the bloodstream. In response, the pancreas releases insulin to help transport glucose from the bloodstream into cells, where it can be used for energy or stored for later use.

Importance of Nutrition in Diabetes Management

Nutrition plays a critical role in managing diabetes by helping to control blood sugar levels, maintain a healthy weight, and reduce the risk of complications. A well-balanced diet can also improve overall health and well-being. By making healthy food choices and managing portion sizes, individuals with diabetes can better control their condition and reduce the need for medication.

Basics of a Diabetic-Friendly Diet

Crafting a diabetic-friendly diet involves understanding how different foods affect blood sugar levels and making choices that promote stable glucose levels. Key principles of a diabetic-friendly diet include:

Balancing Macronutrients (Carbohydrates, Protein, Fat)

Carbohydrates, protein, and fat are the three main macronutrients that provide energy and essential nutrients. Balancing these macronutrients can help prevent spikes in blood sugar levels and promote overall health.

- **Carbohydrates**: Carbohydrates have the most significant impact on blood sugar levels because they are broken down into glucose during digestion. However, not all carbohydrates are created equal. Focus on consuming complex carbohydrates, such as whole grains, fruits, vegetables, and legumes, which are digested more slowly and have less of an impact on blood sugar levels compared to simple carbohydrates like refined grains and sugary foods.

- **Protein**: Including protein-rich foods, such as lean meats, poultry, fish, tofu, eggs, and dairy products, in your meals can help stabilize blood sugar levels and promote satiety. Protein also plays a crucial role in muscle repair and maintenance.

- **Fat**: While fats are high in calories, they can be part of a healthy diabetic-friendly diet when consumed in moderation. Choose healthy fats, such as those found in nuts, seeds, avocados, and olive oil, which can help improve insulin sensitivity and reduce the risk of heart disease.

Glycemic Index and Its Impact on Blood Sugar

The glycemic index (GI) is a ranking system that measures how quickly carbohydrates in food raise blood sugar levels. Foods with a high GI are rapidly digested and cause a sharp increase in blood sugar levels, while foods with a low GI are digested more slowly, resulting in a gradual rise in blood sugar levels.

Portion Control and Meal Timing

In addition to choosing the right types of foods, portion control and meal timing are essential aspects of managing blood sugar levels. Eating regular, balanced meals and snacks throughout the day can help prevent blood sugar spikes and crashes. Aim for smaller, more frequent meals and avoid skipping meals, which can lead to overeating and instability in blood sugar levels.

Reading Food Labels and Making Smart Choices

Understanding how to read food labels can empower individuals with diabetes to make informed choices and better manage their condition. Key points to consider when reading food labels include:

Understanding Nutrition Labels

Nutrition labels provide valuable information about the nutrient content of packaged foods, including serving size, calories, macronutrients, vitamins, and minerals. Pay attention to portion sizes and serving sizes to ensure you are consuming appropriate amounts of nutrients.

Identifying Hidden Sugars and Carbohydrates

Many processed and packaged foods contain hidden sugars and carbohydrates, which can quickly add up and lead to blood sugar spikes. Be mindful of ingredients such as high-fructose corn syrup, maltose, dextrose, and sucrose, as well as hidden sources of carbohydrates like white flour and refined grains.

Choosing Nutrient-Dense Foods

Opting for nutrient-dense foods can help ensure you are getting essential vitamins, minerals, and antioxidants without excess calories or added sugars. Focus on incorporating a variety of colorful fruits and vegetables, whole grains, lean proteins, and healthy fats into your diet to support overall health and well-being.

In conclusion, understanding the relationship between diabetes and nutrition is essential for effectively managing the condition and reducing the risk of complications. By following a diabetic-friendly diet that emphasizes balanced macronutrients, low-glycemic foods, portion control, and smart food choices, individuals with diabetes can better control their blood sugar levels and improve their overall quality of life. Regular monitoring of blood sugar levels, along with guidance from healthcare professionals, can further support diabetes management efforts and promote long-term health and well-being.

CHAPTER TWO

Essential Cooking Techniques for Diabetics

Cooking plays a pivotal role in managing diabetes as it directly influences the nutritional content and overall healthiness of meals. This section will explore essential cooking techniques tailored for individuals with diabetes, focusing on healthy cooking methods, flavorful seasoning and spices, and smart substitutions in recipes to promote blood sugar control and overall well-being.

Healthy Cooking Methods

Choosing the right cooking methods can help retain nutrients while minimizing added fats and sugars, making meals healthier for individuals with diabetes. Here are some healthy cooking techniques to consider:

Grilling and Broiling

Grilling and broiling are excellent methods for cooking lean meats, poultry, fish, and vegetables without adding extra fats. These techniques involve cooking food over direct heat, allowing excess fat to drip away, resulting in flavorful and nutritious dishes.

Baking and Roasting

Baking and roasting are low-fat cooking methods that require little to no added oil or fat. By cooking food in the oven, you can achieve a crispy exterior and tender interior without compromising on flavor. These methods are particularly suitable for vegetables, poultry, and fish.

Sauteing and Stir-Frying

Sauteing and stir-frying involve cooking food quickly over high heat with minimal oil. These techniques are ideal for preserving the natural flavors and textures of ingredients while reducing the need for added fats. Use heart-healthy oils like olive oil or avocado oil sparingly to enhance flavor.

Flavorful Seasoning and Spices

Enhancing the taste of dishes with herbs, spices, and seasonings can elevate the flavor profile without adding extra salt, sugar, or unhealthy fats. Here are some flavorful options to consider:

Salt-Free Seasonings

Experiment with salt-free seasonings like garlic powder, onion powder, black pepper, chili powder, cumin, and paprika to add depth and complexity to your meals without increasing sodium intake. Look for sodium-free seasoning blends at your local grocery store or create your own custom blends at home.

Fresh Herbs and Citrus Zest

Fresh herbs, such as basil, parsley, cilantro, and thyme, add vibrant flavors and aromas to dishes without extra calories or carbohydrates. Similarly, citrus zest from lemons, limes, and oranges can provide a burst of freshness and acidity to savory and sweet recipes.

Spice Blends and Marinades

Create homemade spice blends and marinades using a variety of herbs, spices, citrus juices, and vinegar to infuse flavor into meats, poultry, fish, and vegetables. Avoid pre-packaged marinades and seasoning mixes, which often contain added sugars and unhealthy additives.

Smart Substitutions in Recipes

Making smart ingredient substitutions in recipes can help reduce the overall carbohydrate, sugar, and fat content of dishes while maintaining flavor and texture. Consider the following substitutions to make your recipes more diabetes-friendly:

Using Whole Grain Flours and Pasta

Swap refined flours and pasta with whole grain alternatives like whole wheat flour, oat flour, almond flour, and whole grain pasta. These options are higher in fiber and nutrients, which can help stabilize blood sugar levels and promote satiety.

Swapping Sugars with Natural Sweeteners

Replace refined sugars with natural sweeteners like stevia, erythritol, monk fruit extract, or xylitol to sweeten recipes without causing spikes in blood sugar levels. These sweeteners are lower in calories and carbohydrates and have minimal impact on blood glucose levels.

Substituting High-Fat Ingredients with Healthier Options

Replace high-fat ingredients like butter, cream, and full-fat dairy with healthier alternatives such as olive oil, Greek yogurt, avocado, and coconut milk. These substitutions can help reduce saturated fat intake while adding flavor and richness to dishes.

In conclusion, incorporating essential cooking techniques tailored for individuals with diabetes can help improve blood sugar control and overall health outcomes. By choosing healthy cooking methods, flavorful seasonings and spices, and smart substitutions in recipes, individuals with diabetes can enjoy delicious and nutritious meals that support their dietary needs and promote well-being. Experiment with different ingredients and flavor combinations to discover new culinary favorites while managing diabetes effectively.

CHAPTER THREE

Quick and Easy Diabetic Breakfasts

For individuals with diabetes, starting the day with a nutritious breakfast is essential for maintaining stable blood sugar levels and providing energy for the day ahead. This section will present a variety of quick and easy diabetic breakfast ideas, including energizing smoothie recipes, simple oatmeal variations, and balanced breakfast plates to kickstart your morning on the right foot.

Energizing Smoothie Recipes

Smoothies are a convenient and delicious way to pack a variety of nutrients into a single meal. Here are some energizing smoothie recipes that are low in added sugars and high in fiber, protein, and healthy fats:

Green Breakfast Smoothie

Ingredients:

- 1 cup spinach
- 1/2 cup kale
- 1/2 banana (frozen for creaminess)
- 1/4 avocado
- 1/2 cup unsweetened almond milk
- 1 tablespoon chia seeds
- Ice cubes (optional)

Instructions:

1. Combine all ingredients in a blender.

2. Blend until smooth and creamy.

3. Pour into a glass and enjoy immediately.

Berry Blast Smoothie Bowl

Ingredients:

- 1/2 cup mixed berries (such as strawberries, blueberries, and raspberries)

- 1/2 banana (frozen for creaminess)

- 1/2 cup plain Greek yogurt

- 1 tablespoon almond butter

- 1/4 cup unsweetened almond milk

- Toppings: sliced almonds, shredded coconut, chia seeds

Instructions:

1. In a blender, combine the mixed berries, banana, Greek yogurt, almond butter, and almond milk.

2. Blend until smooth and creamy.

3. Pour the smoothie into a bowl and top with sliced almonds, shredded coconut, and chia seeds.

4. Enjoy with a spoon!

Protein-Packed Peanut Butter Smoothie

Ingredients:

- 1 tablespoon natural peanut butter
- 1/2 banana
- 1 scoop vanilla protein powder
- 1 cup unsweetened almond milk
- Ice cubes (optional)

Instructions:

1. In a blender, combine the peanut butter, banana, protein powder, and almond milk.
2. Blend until smooth and creamy.
3. Add ice cubes if desired and blend again until well combined.
4. Pour into a glass and enjoy!

Simple Oatmeal Variations

Oatmeal is a versatile and nutritious breakfast option that can be customized with a variety of toppings and flavorings. Here are some simple oatmeal variations to try:

Overnight Oats with Fruit and Nuts

Ingredients:

- 1/2 cup old-fashioned oats

- 1/2 cup unsweetened almond milk

- 1/4 cup Greek yogurt

- 1/2 banana, mashed

- 1 tablespoon chia seeds

- Toppings: sliced strawberries, chopped nuts, drizzle of honey (optional)

Instructions:

1. In a jar or bowl, combine the oats, almond milk, Greek yogurt, mashed banana, and chia seeds.

2. Stir well to combine.

3. Cover and refrigerate overnight.

4. In the morning, top with sliced strawberries, chopped nuts, and a drizzle of honey if desired.

5. Enjoy cold or warm it up in the microwave before serving.

Savory Oatmeal with Spinach and Cheese

Ingredients:

- 1/2 cup old-fashioned oats

- 1 cup water or low-sodium vegetable broth

- Handful of fresh spinach

- 1/4 cup shredded cheese (such as cheddar or feta)

- Salt and pepper to taste

Instructions:

1. In a saucepan, bring the water or vegetable broth to a boil.

2. Stir in the oats and reduce the heat to low.

3. Cook for 5-7 minutes, stirring occasionally, until the oats are tender and the liquid is absorbed.

4. Stir in the spinach until wilted.

5. Remove from heat and stir in the shredded cheese until melted.

6. Season with salt and pepper to taste.

7. Serve hot and enjoy!

Baked Oatmeal Cups with Berries

Ingredients:

- 2 cups old-fashioned oats

- 1 teaspoon baking powder

- 1/2 teaspoon cinnamon

- 1/4 teaspoon salt

- 1 cup unsweetened almond milk

- 1/4 cup pure maple syrup

- 1 egg

- 1 teaspoon vanilla extract

- 1 cup mixed berries (such as blueberries, raspberries, and strawberries)

Instructions:

1. Preheat the oven to 350°F (175°C). Grease a muffin tin or line with paper liners.

2. In a large bowl, combine the oats, baking powder, cinnamon, and salt.

3. In a separate bowl, whisk together the almond milk, maple syrup, egg, and vanilla extract.

4. Pour the wet ingredients into the dry ingredients and stir until well combined.

5. Gently fold in the mixed berries.

6. Divide the oat mixture evenly among the muffin cups.

7. Bake for 20-25 minutes, or until the tops are golden brown and set.

8. Allow the oatmeal cups to cool slightly before serving.

9. Enjoy warm or at room temperature!

Balanced Breakfast Plates

For a more traditional breakfast option, consider assembling a balanced breakfast plate with a combination of protein, carbohydrates, and healthy fats:

Veggie Omelet with Whole Grain Toast

Ingredients:

- 2 eggs

- Handful of diced vegetables (such as bell peppers, onions, spinach, and tomatoes)

- 1 tablespoon shredded cheese (optional)

- 1 slice whole grain bread, toasted

- 1 teaspoon olive oil or cooking spray

- Salt and pepper to taste

Instructions:

1. In a bowl, whisk together the eggs until well beaten.

2. Heat olive oil or cooking spray in a non-stick skillet over medium heat.

3. Add the diced vegetables to the skillet and cook until softened.

4. Pour the beaten eggs over the vegetables, tilting the skillet to distribute evenly.

5. Cook the omelet until the edges start to set, then use a spatula to gently lift and fold the omelet in half.

6. Sprinkle shredded cheese on top if desired.

7. Cook for an additional minute or until the cheese is melted and the eggs are cooked through.

8. Serve the omelet with whole grain toast on the side.

9. Enjoy a nutritious and satisfying breakfast!

Greek Yogurt Parfait with Granola and Berries

Ingredients:

- 1/2 cup plain Greek yogurt

- 1/4 cup granola (choose a low-sugar option)

- 1/4 cup mixed berries (such as strawberries, blueberries, and raspberries)

- Drizzle of honey (optional)

Instructions:

1. In a serving bowl or glass, layer the Greek yogurt, granola, and mixed berries.

2. Repeat the layers until the ingredients are used up.

3. Drizzle honey on top if desired for added sweetness.

4. Serve immediately and enjoy a protein-packed breakfast!

Avocado Toast with Poached Egg and Tomato

Ingredients:

- 1 slice whole grain bread, toasted

- 1/2 avocado, mashed

- 1 poached egg

- Sliced tomato

- Salt and pepper to taste

Instructions:

1. Spread the mashed avocado evenly on top of the toasted whole grain bread.

2. Top with sliced tomato.

3. Carefully place the poached egg on top of the avocado and tomato.

4. Season with salt and pepper to taste.

5. Serve immediately and enjoy a satisfying and nutritious breakfast!

In conclusion, these quick and easy diabetic breakfast ideas offer a variety of options to suit different tastes and preferences. Whether you prefer a refreshing smoothie, a comforting bowl of oatmeal, or a balanced breakfast plate, these recipes are designed to provide sustained energy and support blood sugar control throughout the morning. Experiment with different ingredients and flavor combinations to find your favorite breakfasts that fit seamlessly into your diabetes management plan.

CHAPTER FOUR

Satisfying Diabetic Dinners

Maintaining a balanced and nutritious diet is crucial for managing diabetes effectively. Dinner, in particular, offers an opportunity to enjoy satisfying and flavorful meals that support blood sugar control and overall health. This section presents a variety of diabetic-friendly dinner options, including lean protein entrees, flavorful vegetarian mains, and comforting one-pot meals to help you stay on track with your dietary goals.

Lean Protein Entrees

Incorporating lean protein into your dinner meals can help stabilize blood sugar levels and promote satiety. Here are some delicious and nutritious lean protein entrees to try:

Grilled Salmon with Asparagus and Brown Rice

Ingredients:

- 1 salmon fillet
- 1 bunch asparagus
- 1 cup cooked brown rice
- Olive oil
- Lemon juice
- Salt and pepper to taste

Instructions:

1. Preheat the grill to medium-high heat.
2. Season the salmon fillet with olive oil, lemon juice, salt, and pepper.

3. Place the salmon fillet on the grill and cook for 4-5 minutes on each side, or until cooked through.

4. Meanwhile, toss the asparagus spears with olive oil, salt, and pepper.

5. Grill the asparagus for 2-3 minutes per side, or until tender.

6. Serve the grilled salmon and asparagus with cooked brown rice on the side.

7. Enjoy a delicious and nutritious dinner!

Baked Chicken Breast with Roasted Vegetables

Ingredients:

- 2 chicken breasts

- Assorted vegetables (such as bell peppers, zucchini, and carrots)

- Olive oil

- Garlic powder

- Paprika

- Salt and pepper to taste

Instructions:

1. Preheat the oven to 400°F (200°C).

2. Place the chicken breasts on a baking sheet lined with parchment paper.

3. Drizzle the chicken breasts with olive oil and season with garlic powder, paprika, salt, and pepper.

4. Arrange the assorted vegetables around the chicken breasts on the baking sheet.

5. Drizzle the vegetables with olive oil and season with salt and pepper.

6. Bake in the preheated oven for 20-25 minutes, or until the chicken is cooked through and the vegetables are tender.

7. Serve the baked chicken breast with roasted vegetables for a satisfying and nutritious dinner.

Tofu Stir-Fry with Broccoli and Quinoa

Ingredients:

- 1 block firm tofu, pressed and cubed

- 2 cups broccoli florets

- 1 bell pepper, sliced

- 1 carrot, sliced

- 1 cup cooked quinoa

- Stir-fry sauce (soy sauce, garlic, ginger, sesame oil)

- Olive oil

Instructions:

1. Heat olive oil in a large skillet or wok over medium-high heat.

2. Add the cubed tofu to the skillet and cook until golden brown on all sides.

3. Remove the tofu from the skillet and set aside.

4. In the same skillet, add a little more olive oil if needed, then add the broccoli, bell pepper, and carrot.

5. Stir-fry the vegetables until crisp-tender.

6. Return the tofu to the skillet and add the cooked quinoa.

7. Pour the stir-fry sauce over the tofu, vegetables, and quinoa, and toss to coat evenly.

8. Cook for an additional 2-3 minutes, or until heated through.

9. Serve the tofu stir-fry with broccoli and quinoa for a flavorful and satisfying dinner option.

Flavorful Vegetarian Mains

Vegetarian meals can be just as satisfying and flavorful as their meat-based counterparts. Here are some delicious and nutritious vegetarian main dishes to enjoy:

Eggplant Parmesan with Whole Wheat Pasta

Ingredients:

- 1 large eggplant, sliced

- Whole wheat pasta

- Marinara sauce

- Mozzarella cheese

- Parmesan cheese

- Olive oil

- Salt and pepper to taste

Instructions:

1. Preheat the oven to 375°F (190°C).

2. Place the eggplant slices on a baking sheet lined with parchment paper.

3. Brush the eggplant slices with olive oil and season with salt and pepper.

4. Bake in the preheated oven for 15-20 minutes, or until tender and golden brown.

5. Meanwhile, cook the whole wheat pasta according to package instructions.

6. In a baking dish, layer marinara sauce, eggplant slices, mozzarella cheese, and Parmesan cheese.

7. Repeat the layers until all ingredients are used up, ending with a layer of cheese on top.

8. Bake in the oven for an additional 20-25 minutes, or until the cheese is melted and bubbly.

9. Serve the eggplant Parmesan with whole wheat pasta for a satisfying and hearty vegetarian meal.

Lentil Curry with Cauliflower Rice

Ingredients:

- 1 cup dried lentils

- 1 onion, chopped

- 2 cloves garlic, minced

- 1 tablespoon curry powder

- 1 can coconut milk

- 1 head cauliflower

- Olive oil

- Salt and pepper to taste

Instructions:

1. Cook the lentils according to package instructions until tender.

2. In a large skillet, heat olive oil over medium heat.

3. Add the chopped onion and minced garlic to the skillet and cook until softened.

4. Stir in the curry powder and cook for an additional minute.

5. Add the cooked lentils and coconut milk to the skillet, and simmer for 10-15 minutes, or until heated through and thickened.

6. Meanwhile, prepare the cauliflower rice by pulsing cauliflower florets in a food processor until they resemble rice.

7. Heat a little olive oil in a separate skillet over medium heat.

8. Add the cauliflower rice to the skillet and cook for 5-7 minutes, or until tender.

9. Season the cauliflower rice with salt and pepper to taste.

10.   Serve the lentil curry with cauliflower rice for a flavorful and nutritious vegetarian dinner.

Stuffed Bell Peppers with Black Beans and Corn

Ingredients:

- 4 bell peppers, halved and seeds removed

- 1 can black beans, drained and rinsed

- 1 cup corn kernels (fresh or frozen)

- 1 cup cooked quinoa

- 1 cup salsa

- Shredded cheese (optional)

- Olive oil

- Salt and pepper to taste

Instructions:

1. Preheat the oven to 375°F (190°C).

2. Place the bell pepper halves in a baking dish.

3. In a large bowl, combine the black beans, corn kernels, cooked quinoa, salsa, olive oil, salt, and pepper.

4. Spoon the black bean mixture into the bell pepper halves until they are filled.

5. If desired, top each stuffed bell pepper with shredded cheese.

6. Cover the baking dish with foil and bake in the preheated oven for 25-30 minutes, or until the peppers are tender.

7. Remove the foil and bake for an additional 5 minutes, or until the cheese is melted and bubbly.

8. Serve the stuffed bell peppers with black beans and corn for a satisfying and colorful vegetarian dinner.

Comforting One-Pot Meals

One-pot meals are convenient and easy to prepare, making them perfect for busy weeknights. Here are some comforting one-pot meal ideas that are sure to please:

Turkey Chili with Beans

Ingredients:

- 1 pound ground turkey
- 1 onion, chopped
- 2 cloves garlic, minced
- 1 can kidney beans, drained and rinsed
- 1 can diced tomatoes
- 1 cup low-sodium chicken broth
- Chili powder, cumin, paprika, salt, and pepper to taste

Instructions:

1. In a large pot or Dutch oven, cook the ground turkey, chopped onion, and minced garlic over medium heat until the turkey is browned and the onion is softened.

2. Stir in the kidney beans, diced tomatoes, chicken broth, and seasonings.

3. Bring the mixture to a boil, then reduce the heat and simmer for 20-30 minutes, stirring occasionally.

4. Taste and adjust the seasonings as needed.

5. Serve the turkey chili hot, garnished with your favorite toppings such as shredded cheese, diced avocado, and chopped cilantro.

Beef and Vegetable Stir-Fry with Brown Rice

Ingredients:

- 1 pound lean beef, thinly sliced
- Assorted vegetables (such as bell peppers, broccoli, carrots, and snap peas)
- Low-sodium soy sauce
- Garlic, minced
- Ginger, grated
- Olive oil
- Cooked brown rice

Instructions:

1. In a large skillet or wok, heat olive oil over high heat.

2. Add the thinly sliced beef to the skillet and cook until browned.

3. Remove the beef from the skillet and set aside.

4. In the same skillet, add a little more olive oil if needed, then add the minced garlic and grated ginger.

5. Stir-fry the assorted vegetables until crisp-tender.

6. Return the cooked beef to the skillet and add low-sodium soy sauce to taste.

7. Cook for an additional 2-3 minutes, or until heated through.

8. Serve the beef and vegetable stir-fry hot, over cooked brown rice.

Ratatouille with Herbed Quinoa

Ingredients:

- 1 eggplant, diced
- 2 zucchini, diced
- 1 onion, chopped
- 2 bell peppers, diced
- 2 cloves garlic, minced
- 1 can diced tomatoes

- Fresh basil, chopped

- Fresh thyme, chopped

- Olive oil

- Salt and pepper to taste

- Cooked herbed quinoa

Instructions:

1. Heat olive oil in a large pot or Dutch oven over medium heat.

2. Add the chopped onion and minced garlic to the pot and cook until softened.

3. Stir in the diced eggplant, zucchini, bell peppers, diced tomatoes, and chopped herbs.

4. Season with salt and pepper to taste.

5. Cover and simmer for 25-30 minutes, stirring occasionally, until the vegetables are tender.

6. Serve the ratatouille hot, over cooked herbed quinoa.

In conclusion, these satisfying diabetic dinner ideas offer a variety of options to suit different tastes and preferences. Whether you prefer lean protein entrees, flavorful vegetarian mains, or comforting one-pot meals, these recipes are designed to help you enjoy delicious and nutritious dinners while managing your diabetes effectively. Experiment with different ingredients and flavor combinations to find your favorite meals that fit seamlessly into your diabetes management plan.

CHAPTER FIVE

Delicious Diabetic-Friendly Sides

Adding flavorful and nutritious sides to your meals can enhance the dining experience while providing essential nutrients and supporting blood sugar control. This section presents a variety of delicious diabetic-friendly side dishes, including vibrant vegetable dishes, wholesome whole grains, and flavorful bean and legume dishes to complement your main courses.

Vibrant Vegetable Dishes

Incorporating vibrant vegetables into your meals not only adds color and texture but also provides essential vitamins, minerals, and fiber. Here are some delicious vegetable side dish ideas to try:

Roasted Brussels Sprouts with Balsamic Glaze

Ingredients:

- 1 pound Brussels sprouts, trimmed and halved
- 2 tablespoons olive oil
- Salt and pepper to taste
- 2 tablespoons balsamic vinegar
- 1 teaspoon honey (optional)

Instructions:

1. Preheat the oven to 400°F (200°C).
2. In a large bowl, toss the Brussels sprouts with olive oil, salt, and pepper until evenly coated.

3. Spread the Brussels sprouts in a single layer on a baking sheet lined with parchment paper.

4. Roast in the preheated oven for 20-25 minutes, or until tender and caramelized, stirring halfway through.

5. In a small saucepan, heat balsamic vinegar (and honey if using) over medium heat until reduced and thickened, about 5 minutes.

6. Drizzle the roasted Brussels sprouts with the balsamic glaze before serving.

7. Enjoy the flavorful and nutritious side dish!

Steamed Broccoli with Lemon and Garlic

Ingredients:

- 1 head broccoli, cut into florets

- 2 cloves garlic, minced

- Zest of 1 lemon

- Juice of 1/2 lemon

- Olive oil

- Salt and pepper to taste

Instructions:

1. Bring a pot of water to a boil and place a steamer basket over the pot.

2. Add the broccoli florets to the steamer basket and cover with a lid.

3. Steam the broccoli for 4-5 minutes, or until crisp-tender.

4. Meanwhile, heat olive oil in a small skillet over medium heat.

5. Add minced garlic to the skillet and cook until fragrant, about 1 minute.

6. Remove the skillet from heat and stir in lemon zest and lemon juice.

7. Transfer the steamed broccoli to a serving dish and drizzle with the lemon garlic sauce.

8. Season with salt and pepper to taste.

9. Serve the steamed broccoli with lemon and garlic as a refreshing side dish.

Grilled Zucchini and Bell Peppers with Herbs

Ingredients:

- 2 zucchini, sliced

- 2 bell peppers, sliced

- 2 tablespoons olive oil

- Fresh herbs (such as parsley, basil, or thyme)

- Salt and pepper to taste

Instructions:

1. Preheat the grill to medium-high heat.

2. In a large bowl, toss the zucchini and bell peppers with olive oil, salt, and pepper until evenly coated.

3. Place the vegetables on the grill in a single layer.

4. Grill for 3-4 minutes per side, or until tender and lightly charred.

5. Remove the grilled vegetables from the grill and transfer to a serving platter.

6. Sprinkle with fresh herbs before serving.

7. Enjoy the grilled zucchini and bell peppers as a flavorful and nutritious side dish!

Wholesome Whole Grains

Whole grains are rich in fiber, vitamins, and minerals, making them a nutritious addition to any meal. Here are some wholesome whole grain side dish ideas to try:

Quinoa Pilaf with Mixed Vegetables

Ingredients:

- 1 cup quinoa, rinsed

- 2 cups low-sodium vegetable broth

- Assorted vegetables (such as carrots, peas, and bell peppers), diced

- Olive oil

- Garlic powder

- Salt and pepper to taste

Instructions:

1. In a saucepan, bring the vegetable broth to a boil.

2. Add the quinoa to the saucepan and reduce the heat to low.

3. Cover and simmer for 15-20 minutes, or until the quinoa is tender and the liquid is absorbed.

4. Meanwhile, heat olive oil in a skillet over medium heat.

5. Add the diced vegetables to the skillet and sauté until tender.

6. Season the vegetables with garlic powder, salt, and pepper to taste.

7. Fluff the cooked quinoa with a fork and stir in the sautéed vegetables.

8. Serve the quinoa pilaf with mixed vegetables as a wholesome and flavorful side dish.

Brown Rice and Lentil Salad

Ingredients:

- 1 cup brown rice, cooked
- 1 cup cooked lentils
- 1 cucumber, diced
- 1 tomato, diced
- 1/4 cup red onion, finely chopped
- Fresh parsley, chopped
- Lemon juice
- Olive oil
- Salt and pepper to taste

Instructions:

1. In a large bowl, combine the cooked brown rice, cooked lentils, diced cucumber, diced tomato, and chopped red onion.

2. Drizzle with olive oil and lemon juice.

3. Season with salt and pepper to taste.

4. Toss to combine all ingredients.

5. Garnish with fresh parsley before serving.

6. Enjoy the brown rice and lentil salad as a nutritious and satisfying side dish!

Whole Wheat Couscous with Dried Fruit and Almonds

Ingredients:

- 1 cup whole wheat couscous

- 1 1/4 cups low-sodium vegetable broth

- 1/4 cup dried apricots, chopped

- 1/4 cup dried cranberries

- 1/4 cup sliced almonds

- Fresh mint, chopped

- Olive oil

- Salt and pepper to taste

Instructions:

1. In a saucepan, bring the vegetable broth to a boil.

2. Stir in the whole wheat couscous, dried apricots, and dried cranberries.

3. Remove the saucepan from heat, cover, and let stand for 5 minutes.

4. Fluff the couscous with a fork.

5. Drizzle with olive oil and season with salt and pepper to taste.

6. Stir in the sliced almonds and chopped fresh mint.

7. Serve the whole wheat couscous with dried fruit and almonds as a delightful and nutritious side dish.

Flavorful Bean and Legume Dishes

Beans and legumes are excellent sources of plant-based protein, fiber, and essential nutrients. Here are some flavorful bean and legume side dish ideas to incorporate into your meals:

Mediterranean Chickpea Salad

Ingredients:

- 1 can chickpeas, drained and rinsed

- 1 cucumber, diced

- 1 tomato, diced

- 1/4 cup red onion, finely chopped

- Kalamata olives, pitted and sliced

- Feta cheese, crumbled

- Fresh parsley, chopped

- Olive oil

- Lemon juice

- Salt and pepper to taste

Instructions:

1. In a large bowl, combine the chickpeas, diced cucumber, diced tomato, chopped red onion, sliced Kalamata olives, crumbled feta cheese, and chopped fresh parsley.

2. Drizzle with olive oil and lemon juice.

3. Season with salt and pepper to taste.

4. Toss to combine all ingredients.

5. Serve the Mediterranean chickpea salad as a refreshing and flavorful side dish!

Black Bean and Corn Salad with Lime Dressing

Ingredients:

- 1 can black beans, drained and rinsed

- 1 cup corn kernels (fresh or frozen)

- 1 bell pepper, diced

- 1/4 cup red onion, finely chopped

- Fresh cilantro, chopped

- Lime zest and juice

- Olive oil

- Salt and pepper to taste

Instructions:

1. In a large bowl, combine the black beans, corn kernels, diced bell pepper, chopped red onion, and chopped fresh cilantro.

2. In a small bowl, whisk together lime zest, lime juice, olive oil, salt, and pepper to make the dressing.

3. Pour the dressing over the bean and corn mixture.

4. Toss to combine all ingredients.

5. Serve the black bean and corn salad with lime dressing as a zesty and nutritious side dish.

Lentil Soup with Spinach and Tomatoes

Ingredients:

- 1 cup dried lentils

- 4 cups low-sodium vegetable broth

- 1 onion, chopped

- 2 cloves garlic, minced

- 1 can diced tomatoes

- 2 cups fresh spinach leaves

- Olive oil

- Salt and pepper to taste

Instructions:

1. In a large pot, heat olive oil over medium heat.

2. Add the chopped onion and minced garlic to the pot and cook until softened.

3. Add the dried lentils and vegetable broth to the pot.

4. Bring to a boil, then reduce the heat and simmer for 20-25 minutes, or until the lentils are tender.

5. Stir in the diced tomatoes and fresh spinach leaves.

6. Cook for an additional 5 minutes, or until the spinach is wilted.

7. Season with salt and pepper to taste.

8. Serve the lentil soup with spinach and tomatoes as a comforting and nutritious side dish.

In conclusion, these delicious diabetic-friendly side dishes offer a variety of options to add flavor, nutrition, and visual appeal to your meals. Whether you prefer vibrant vegetable dishes, wholesome whole grains, or flavorful bean and legume dishes, these recipes are designed to complement your main courses while supporting your dietary goals and promoting overall well-being. Experiment with different ingredients and flavor combinations to find your favorite sides that fit seamlessly into your diabetes management plan.

CHAPTER SIX

Irresistible Diabetic Desserts

Satisfying your sweet tooth while managing diabetes is possible with these irresistible dessert ideas. From fruity treats to guilt-free baked goods and indulgent dessert swaps, these recipes offer delicious options to enjoy without compromising your health goals.

Fruity Treats and Frozen Delights

1. **Berry and Yogurt Parfait**

   - Ingredients:

     - 1 cup Greek yogurt (unsweetened)

     - 1/2 cup mixed berries (such as strawberries, blueberries, and raspberries)

     - 1 tablespoon honey or maple syrup (optional)

     - Granola for topping (optional)

   - Instructions:

1. In a glass or bowl, layer Greek yogurt, mixed berries, and honey or maple syrup if desired.

2. Repeat the layers until the glass or bowl is filled.

3. Top with granola for added crunch if desired.

4.   Serve immediately or refrigerate until ready to eat.

2. Frozen Banana Bites with Dark Chocolate

- Ingredients:
    - 2 ripe bananas, peeled and sliced into rounds
    - Dark chocolate chips
    - Chopped nuts (optional)
- Instructions:

1.   Place banana slices on a baking sheet lined with parchment paper.

2.   Insert toothpicks into each banana slice.

3.   Melt dark chocolate chips in a microwave-safe bowl in 30-second intervals, stirring until smooth.

4.   Dip each banana slice into the melted chocolate, coating it halfway.

5.   Place the chocolate-coated banana slices back on the baking sheet.

6.   Sprinkle chopped nuts on top if desired.

7.   Freeze for 1-2 hours or until the chocolate is set.

8.   Serve immediately or store in the freezer for a delicious frozen treat.

3. **Mango Sorbet with Fresh Mint**

- Ingredients:

    - 2 ripe mangoes, peeled and diced

    - Fresh mint leaves

    - Lemon juice

    - Honey or agave syrup (optional)

- Instructions:

1. Place diced mangoes in a blender or food processor.

2. Add a few fresh mint leaves and a squeeze of lemon juice.

3. Blend until smooth.

4. Taste the mixture and add honey or agave syrup if additional sweetness is desired.

5. Pour the mixture into a shallow dish and freeze for 4-6 hours, stirring occasionally to prevent ice crystals from forming.

6. Once frozen, scoop the mango sorbet into bowls and garnish with fresh mint leaves.

7. Serve immediately for a refreshing and fruity dessert.

Guilt-Free Baked Goods

4. **Whole Wheat Banana Bread**

- Ingredients:

  - 2 ripe bananas, mashed

  - 1/4 cup unsweetened applesauce

  - 1/4 cup honey or maple syrup

  - 1 egg

  - 1 teaspoon vanilla extract

  - 1 cup whole wheat flour

  - 1 teaspoon baking powder

  - 1/2 teaspoon baking soda

  - 1/2 teaspoon cinnamon

  - Pinch of salt

- Instructions:

1.   Preheat the oven to 350°F (175°C). Grease a loaf pan with cooking spray.

2.   In a mixing bowl, combine mashed bananas, applesauce, honey or maple syrup, egg, and vanilla extract.

3.   In a separate bowl, whisk together whole wheat flour, baking powder, baking soda, cinnamon, and salt.

4.   Gradually add the dry ingredients to the wet ingredients, mixing until just combined.

5.   Pour the batter into the prepared loaf pan.

6.   Bake for 45-50 minutes or until a toothpick inserted into the center comes out clean.

7.   Allow the banana bread to cool in the pan for 10 minutes before transferring it to a wire rack to cool completely.

8.   Slice and enjoy this healthier version of banana bread guilt-free.

5. Almond Flour Chocolate Chip Cookies

- Ingredients:
    - 1 1/2 cups almond flour
    - 1/4 teaspoon baking soda
    - Pinch of salt
    - 1/4 cup coconut oil, melted
    - 1/4 cup honey or maple syrup
    - 1 egg
    - 1 teaspoon vanilla extract
    - 1/2 cup dark chocolate chips

- Instructions:

1. Preheat the oven to 350°F (175°C). Line a baking sheet with parchment paper.

2. In a mixing bowl, whisk together almond flour, baking soda, and salt.

3. In a separate bowl, mix together melted coconut oil, honey or maple syrup, egg, and vanilla extract.

4. Gradually add the dry ingredients to the wet ingredients, mixing until well combined.

5. Fold in dark chocolate chips.

6. Drop tablespoonfuls of dough onto the prepared baking sheet, spacing them 2 inches apart.

7. Flatten each cookie slightly with the back of a spoon.

8. Bake for 10-12 minutes or until golden brown around the edges.

9. Allow the cookies to cool on the baking sheet for 5 minutes before transferring them to a wire rack to cool completely.

10. Enjoy these almond flour chocolate chip cookies as a healthier alternative to traditional cookies.

6. Pumpkin Spice Muffins with Walnuts

- Ingredients:

- 1 1/2 cups whole wheat flour

- 1 teaspoon baking powder

- 1/2 teaspoon baking soda

- 1/2 teaspoon cinnamon

- 1/4 teaspoon nutmeg

- 1/4 teaspoon ginger

- Pinch of cloves

- 1 cup canned pumpkin puree

- 1/2 cup unsweetened applesauce

- 1/4 cup honey or maple syrup

- 1 egg

- 1 teaspoon vanilla extract

- 1/2 cup chopped walnuts

- Instructions:

1.   Preheat the oven to 350°F (175°C). Line a muffin tin with paper liners.

2.   In a mixing bowl, whisk together whole wheat flour, baking powder, baking soda, cinnamon, nutmeg, ginger, and cloves.

3. In a separate bowl, mix together pumpkin puree, applesauce, honey or maple syrup, egg, and vanilla extract.

4. Gradually add the dry ingredients to the wet ingredients, mixing until just combined.

5. Fold in chopped walnuts.

6. Divide the batter evenly among the prepared muffin cups.

7. Bake for 20-25 minutes or until a toothpick inserted into the center comes out clean.

8. Allow the muffins to cool in the tin for 5 minutes before transferring them to a wire rack to cool completely.

9. Enjoy these pumpkin spice muffins as a delicious and nutritious treat.

Indulgent Dessert Swaps

7. Avocado Chocolate Pudding

- Ingredients:
  - 2 ripe avocados
  - 1/4 cup cocoa powder
  - 1/4 cup honey or maple syrup
  - 1 teaspoon vanilla extract
  - Pinch of salt

- Fresh berries for serving

- Instructions:

1. Scoop the flesh of the avocados into a blender or food processor.

2. Add cocoa powder, honey or maple syrup, vanilla extract, and salt.

3. Blend until smooth and creamy, scraping down the sides of the blender or food processor as needed.

4. Divide the avocado chocolate pudding into serving dishes.

5. Chill in the refrigerator for at least 30 minutes before serving.

6. Garnish with fresh berries before serving for added freshness and flavor.

8. **Greek Yogurt Cheesecake with Berry Compote**

- Ingredients:

  - 1 1/2 cups Greek yogurt

  - 1/4 cup honey or maple syrup

  - 1 egg

  - 1 teaspoon vanilla extract

  - Graham cracker crust (store-bought or homemade)

- Fresh berries for garnish

- For the berry compote:

    - 1 cup mixed berries (such as strawberries, blueberries, and raspberries)

    - 1 tablespoon honey or maple syrup

    - 1 tablespoon lemon juice

- Instructions:

1. Preheat the oven to 325°F (160°C). Grease a 9-inch springform pan and line the bottom with parchment paper.

2. In a mixing bowl, whisk together Greek yogurt, honey or maple syrup, egg, and vanilla extract until smooth.

3. Pour the yogurt mixture into the prepared graham cracker crust.

4. Bake for 25-30 minutes or until the center is set.

5. Allow the cheesecake to cool completely in the pan, then refrigerate for at least 4 hours or overnight.

6. Meanwhile, prepare the berry compote by combining mixed berries, honey or maple syrup, and lemon juice in a saucepan.

7. Cook over medium heat until the berries break down and the mixture thickens, stirring occasionally.

8.   Let the berry compote cool before serving.

9.   Serve slices of Greek yogurt cheesecake with berry compote and fresh berries for a delightful dessert.

9. **Coconut Milk Rice Pudding with Cinnamon**

- Ingredients:
    - 1 cup white rice
    - 2 cups coconut milk
    - 1/4 cup honey or maple syrup
    - 1 teaspoon vanilla extract
    - Pinch of salt
    - Ground cinnamon for garnish
- Instructions:

1.   In a saucepan, combine white rice, coconut milk, honey or maple syrup, vanilla extract, and salt.

2.   Bring the mixture to a boil, then reduce the heat to low and simmer, covered, for 20-25 minutes or until the rice is cooked and the mixture is creamy, stirring occasionally.

3.   Remove from heat and let the rice pudding cool slightly.

4.   Divide the rice pudding into serving bowls.

5.   Sprinkle ground cinnamon on top for added flavor and garnish.

6.   Serve the coconut milk rice pudding warm or chilled for a comforting and indulgent dessert.

In conclusion, these irresistible diabetic desserts offer a variety of options to satisfy your sweet cravings while managing your blood sugar levels effectively. Whether you prefer fruity treats and frozen delights, guilt-free baked goods, or indulgent dessert swaps, these recipes are designed to provide delicious and satisfying options that fit seamlessly into your diabetes management plan. Enjoy these desserts in moderation as part of a balanced diet and healthy lifestyle.

CHAPTER EIGHT

Diabetic-Friendly Snacks for Anytime

Keeping your blood sugar levels stable throughout the day is essential for managing diabetes. These diabetic-friendly snacks offer a combination of nutrients to keep you feeling satisfied and energized without causing spikes in blood sugar levels. From nutritious nuts and seeds to veggie snacks and dips, and fruit-based treats, these snack ideas are perfect for anytime cravings.

Nutritious Nuts and Seeds

1. **Almonds, Walnuts, and Pistachios**

   - Nuts are packed with healthy fats, protein, and fiber, making them an excellent snack choice for diabetes management. Almonds, walnuts, and pistachios are particularly beneficial due to their nutrient content.

   - Portion control is key when enjoying nuts as they are calorie-dense. Aim for a small handful (about 1 ounce) per serving to avoid overeating.

2. **Pumpkin Seeds and Sunflower Seeds**

   - Pumpkin seeds and sunflower seeds are rich in protein, healthy fats, and essential minerals like magnesium and zinc.

- Sprinkle pumpkin seeds or sunflower seeds on salads, yogurt, or oatmeal for added crunch and nutrition.

3. Trail Mix with Dried Fruit

- Create your own trail mix by combining a variety of nuts, seeds, and dried fruit such as almonds, cashews, pumpkin seeds, sunflower seeds, dried cranberries, and raisins.

- Be mindful of portion sizes and choose unsweetened dried fruits to minimize added sugars.

Veggie Snacks and Dips

1. Carrot Sticks with Hummus

- Carrot sticks are low in calories and high in fiber, making them a satisfying snack choice. Pair them with hummus for added protein and flavor.

- Opt for homemade or store-bought hummus without added sugars and artificial ingredients.

2. Celery Sticks with Peanut Butter

- Celery sticks are crunchy and refreshing, perfect for snacking. Spread peanut butter (or almond butter) on celery sticks for a combination of protein and fiber.

- Choose natural peanut butter without added sugars or hydrogenated oils.

3. Cucumber Slices with Greek Yogurt Dip

- Cucumber slices are hydrating and low in calories, making them an excellent snack option. Dip cucumber slices in Greek yogurt seasoned with herbs and spices for added protein and flavor.

- Greek yogurt provides probiotics and protein while keeping the dip creamy and satisfying.

Fruit-Based Treats

1. Apple Slices with Almond Butter

- Apples are a good source of fiber and antioxidants, while almond butter provides healthy fats and protein. Spread almond butter on apple slices for a sweet and satisfying snack.

- Choose crunchy apples like Granny Smith or Fuji for a refreshing crunch.

2. Mixed Berries with Cottage Cheese

- Berries such as strawberries, blueberries, and raspberries are low in calories and high in fiber and antioxidants. Pair mixed berries with cottage cheese for a protein-rich snack that will keep you feeling full.

- Opt for low-fat or plain Greek yogurt for added protein and creaminess.

3. Frozen Grapes or Banana Slices

- Frozen grapes or banana slices make for a refreshing and naturally sweet snack. Simply freeze grapes or banana slices and enjoy them straight from the freezer.

- Frozen fruits can satisfy your sweet cravings while providing essential vitamins, minerals, and fiber.

These diabetic-friendly snacks offer a balance of nutrients to support your health and help manage blood sugar levels. Incorporate these snacks into your daily routine to keep hunger at bay and maintain energy levels throughout the day. Remember to practice portion control and choose whole, unprocessed foods whenever possible for optimal nutrition.

CHAPTER NINE

Dining Out and Socializing with Diabetes

Managing diabetes doesn't mean you have to miss out on dining out or socializing with friends and family. With a little planning and awareness, you can enjoy meals at restaurants, navigate special occasions, and even travel while keeping your blood sugar levels in check. Here's how to make the most of these social situations while prioritizing your health.

Making Healthy Choices at Restaurants

1. **Reviewing Menus in Advance**

   - Before heading to a restaurant, take some time to review the menu online if possible. Look for dishes that are grilled, steamed, or baked, as these cooking methods tend to be lower in added fats and sugars.

   - Pay attention to portion sizes and consider ordering appetizers or sharing a main course to control your portion sizes.

2. **Opting for Grilled or Steamed Options**

   - When ordering at the restaurant, choose grilled, baked, or steamed dishes over fried or breaded options. Grilled fish or chicken, steamed vegetables, and salads with lean protein are usually good choices.

   - Ask for sauces, dressings, and condiments on the side to control the amount you consume, or request substitutions for healthier options.

3. **Requesting Modifications**

   - Don't be afraid to ask for modifications to suit your dietary needs. Requesting items to be cooked without added fats or sauces, substituting side dishes for steamed vegetables or salad, or asking for whole grain options can help you make healthier choices.

Enjoying Special Occasions

1. **Bringing a Dish to Share**

   - If you're attending a social gathering or potluck, consider bringing a dish that fits your dietary preferences and needs. This ensures that you have a healthier option to enjoy while still participating in the festivities.

   - Choose dishes that are rich in vegetables, lean proteins, and whole grains, such as salads, vegetable platters with hummus, or grilled skewers.

2. **Moderating Alcohol Consumption**

   - Alcohol can affect blood sugar levels and may interact with diabetes medications. If you choose to drink, do so in moderation and opt for lower-sugar options like light beer, dry wine, or spirits mixed with sugar-free mixers.

   - Be mindful of portion sizes and aim to stay hydrated by alternating alcoholic beverages with water or other non-caloric drinks.

3. **Choosing Desserts Wisely**

- When indulging in desserts, opt for lighter options such as fresh fruit, sorbet, or a small portion of a lower-sugar dessert. Sharing desserts with others can also help you enjoy a taste without overindulging.

- Consider asking for a fruit plate or a coffee with a splash of cream instead of a traditional dessert to satisfy your sweet tooth without causing a spike in blood sugar levels.

Traveling with Diabetes

1. Packing Snacks and Medications

- When traveling, be sure to pack snacks and medications to manage your blood sugar levels. Portable options like nuts, seeds, whole fruit, or protein bars can help keep hunger at bay between meals.

- Carry your diabetes medications, blood glucose monitor, and emergency supplies in your carry-on luggage to ensure they're easily accessible during your journey.

2. Adapting to Local Cuisine

- Embrace the local cuisine but make mindful choices to keep your blood sugar levels stable. Look for dishes that incorporate lean proteins, whole grains, and plenty of vegetables, and be cautious of portion sizes.

- Opt for grilled, steamed, or roasted dishes over fried or heavily processed options, and be mindful of added sugars and sauces in traditional dishes.

3. **Staying Active and Hydrated**

- Maintain your regular exercise routine as much as possible while traveling to help regulate blood sugar levels and manage stress.

- Stay hydrated by drinking plenty of water throughout your journey, especially if you're flying or visiting warmer climates. Carry a reusable water bottle with you to stay hydrated on the go.

By making informed choices, planning ahead, and advocating for your dietary needs, you can enjoy dining out, socializing with friends and family, and traveling while effectively managing your diabetes. Remember to listen to your body, monitor your blood sugar levels regularly, and seek support from healthcare professionals if needed to ensure your well-being while enjoying life to the fullest.

CHAPTER TEN

Long-Term Strategies for Diabetes Management

Effectively managing diabetes requires a comprehensive approach that encompasses lifestyle changes, regular monitoring, and ongoing support. By implementing long-term strategies, individuals with diabetes can achieve better health outcomes and improve their quality of life. Here are key strategies for long-term diabetes management:

Setting Realistic Goals

1. Establishing Healthy Habits

- Set achievable goals for adopting healthy lifestyle habits such as maintaining a balanced diet, engaging in regular physical activity, and managing stress effectively.

- Start with small, manageable changes and gradually incorporate new habits into your daily routine. Celebrate each milestone as you progress toward your long-term goals.

2. Monitoring Blood Sugar Levels

- Regularly monitor your blood sugar levels as directed by your healthcare provider. Keep track of your readings and identify patterns to better understand how your lifestyle choices and medication regimen impact your blood glucose levels.

- Use blood glucose monitoring devices, continuous glucose monitors (CGMs), or smartphone apps to track your blood sugar levels conveniently.

3. Celebrating Successes

- Celebrate your achievements and milestones along your diabetes management journey. Whether it's reaching a target blood sugar level, losing weight, or consistently following your treatment plan, acknowledge your progress and reward yourself for your efforts.

Building a Support System

1. Connecting with Healthcare Providers

- Establish a strong partnership with your healthcare team, including your primary care physician, endocrinologist, diabetes educator, and other specialists. Work collaboratively to develop a personalized diabetes management plan tailored to your individual needs and goals.

- Schedule regular check-ups and screenings to monitor your overall health, assess your diabetes management progress, and make any necessary adjustments to your treatment plan.

2. Seeking Support from Friends and Family

- Share your diabetes journey with trusted friends and family members who can provide emotional support and encouragement. Educate them about diabetes management and how they can support you in making healthy lifestyle choices.

- Communicate your needs and concerns openly with your loved ones, and involve them in your diabetes management plan to foster a supportive environment.

3. Joining Diabetes Support Groups

- Connect with others who are living with diabetes by joining local or online support groups. These communities provide a valuable source of empathy, shared experiences, and practical advice from peers who understand the challenges of managing diabetes.

- Participate in support group meetings, educational events, and online forums to gain insights, exchange tips, and build friendships with fellow individuals with diabetes.

Prioritizing Self-Care

1. Managing Stress

- Practice stress management techniques such as deep breathing exercises, meditation, yoga, or mindfulness to reduce stress levels and promote emotional well-being.

- Identify stress triggers and develop coping strategies to effectively manage stress in your daily life. Engage in activities that bring you joy and relaxation, such as hobbies, spending time in nature, or listening to music.

2. Getting Regular Exercise

- Incorporate regular physical activity into your routine to improve insulin sensitivity, lower blood sugar levels, and support overall health. Aim for at least 150 minutes of moderate-intensity aerobic exercise per week, such as brisk walking, cycling, swimming, or dancing.

- Include strength training exercises two to three times per week to build muscle mass, improve metabolism, and enhance cardiovascular health.

3. Getting Enough Sleep

- Prioritize adequate sleep and establish a consistent sleep schedule to support optimal health and diabetes management. Aim for seven to nine hours of quality sleep each night to allow your body to rest, repair, and regulate hormones.

- Create a relaxing bedtime routine, avoid caffeine and electronic devices before bedtime, and create a comfortable sleep environment to promote restful sleep.

By implementing these long-term strategies for diabetes management, individuals can take proactive steps to control their blood sugar levels, prevent complications, and improve their overall health and well-being. Consistency, support, and self-care are essential components of successful diabetes management for the long term.

The Flex Diet:

Definition:

The Flex Diet, developed by James Beckerman, MD, is a flexible and customizable approach to weight loss and healthy living. It emphasizes the importance of flexibility, balance, and individualization in dietary choices, exercise routines, and lifestyle habits. The diet encourages participants to "flex" their approach to eating and fitness based on personal preferences, goals, and lifestyle factors. It offers practical strategies for making healthier choices, incorporating physical activity, managing stress, and building sustainable habits for long-term success.

Ingredients:

- Fruits: Berries, apples, oranges, bananas, mangoes, melons, etc.

- Vegetables: Leafy greens, broccoli, cauliflower, bell peppers, carrots, onions, etc.

- Whole Grains: Brown rice, quinoa, oats, barley, whole wheat bread, whole grain pasta.

- Lean Proteins: Chicken, turkey, fish, seafood, tofu, tempeh, lean cuts of beef or pork.

- Healthy Fats: Avocado, nuts, seeds, olive oil.

- Low-Fat Dairy Products: Greek yogurt, cottage cheese, skim milk.

Instructions/How to Prepare:

1. Determine personal health and wellness goals, considering factors such as weight loss, fitness, energy levels, and overall well-being.

2. Evaluate current eating habits, exercise routines, and lifestyle behaviors to identify areas for improvement and opportunities for change.

3. Experiment with different dietary approaches, such as Mediterranean, plant-based, low-carb, or intermittent fasting, to find what works best for individual preferences and needs.

4. Focus on consuming a balanced and varied diet that includes a wide variety of nutrient-rich foods such as fruits, vegetables, whole grains, lean proteins, and healthy fats.

5. Practice portion control and mindful eating by listening to hunger and fullness cues, eating slowly, and savoring each bite.

6. Incorporate regular physical activity into daily routines, including cardiovascular exercise, strength training, flexibility exercises, and recreational activities that are enjoyable and sustainable.

7. Manage stress and prioritize self-care by practicing relaxation techniques, mindfulness, meditation, and other stress-reducing activities.

8. Be flexible and adaptable in making dietary and lifestyle changes, recognizing that progress may not always be linear and that setbacks are part of the journey.

9. Seek support from friends, family, or a health coach for accountability, encouragement, and motivation throughout the process.

10. Embrace a lifelong commitment to health and wellness, continually reassessing goals, making adjustments as needed, and celebrating successes along the way.

Nutrisystem:

Definition:

Nutrisystem is a commercial weight loss program that offers pre-packaged meals and snacks delivered directly to customers' homes. The program aims to simplify weight loss by providing portion-controlled, calorie- and nutrient-balanced meals that require minimal preparation. Nutrisystem offers several plans tailored to different dietary preferences and weight loss goals, including basic, core, vegetarian, and diabetic-friendly options. The program also includes support tools such as counseling, online resources, and a mobile app to help participants track progress and stay motivated.

Ingredients:

- Pre-Packaged Meals: Breakfasts, lunches, dinners, and snacks formulated to meet specific calorie and nutritional targets.

- Variety of Foods: Nutrisystem meals and snacks include a range of options such as pasta dishes, pizzas, burgers, soups, salads, and desserts.

- Fruits and Vegetables: Participants are encouraged to supplement Nutrisystem meals with fresh fruits, vegetables, and salads for added fiber, vitamins, and minerals.

- Flex Meals: Nutrisystem offers flexibility with "flex meals," allowing participants to prepare their meals using guidelines provided by the program.

- Snacks: Nutrisystem provides snacks such as bars, shakes, and cookies to help curb hunger between meals.

Instructions/How to Prepare:

1. Choose a Nutrisystem plan based on individual weight loss goals, dietary preferences, and budget.

2. Receive pre-packaged meals and snacks delivered to your doorstep, following the Nutrisystem meal plan and eating schedule.

3. Enjoy Nutrisystem meals and snacks as directed, incorporating fresh fruits, vegetables, and salads as recommended for added nutrition and variety.

4. Supplement Nutrisystem meals with water or other non-caloric beverages to stay hydrated throughout the day.

5. Utilize support tools such as counseling, online resources, and the Nutrisystem app to track progress, access meal plans, and receive personalized guidance and support.

6. Incorporate physical activity into daily routines to complement Nutrisystem's weight loss program and promote overall health and well-being.

7. Practice portion control and mindful eating by savoring each bite and paying attention to hunger and fullness cues.

8. Monitor weight loss progress and adjust Nutrisystem meal plans as needed to achieve and maintain desired results.

9. Continue following Nutrisystem's maintenance plan and lifestyle recommendations to sustain weight loss and promote long-term success.

10.   Seek support from the Nutrisystem community, including counselors, fellow participants, and online forums, for motivation, encouragement, and accountability throughout the weight loss journey.

Jenny Craig:

Definition:

Jenny Craig is a commercial weight loss program that combines pre-packaged meals and personalized coaching to help individuals achieve their weight loss goals. The program offers a variety of meal plans tailored to different dietary preferences, including standard, vegetarian, and gluten-free options. Participants receive pre-portioned meals and snacks delivered to their homes or can pick them up at Jenny Craig centers. In addition to meal delivery, Jenny Craig provides one-on-one coaching, support tools, and online resources to help clients develop healthy habits, overcome obstacles, and achieve long-term success.

Ingredients:

- Pre-Packaged Meals: Breakfasts, lunches, dinners, and snacks formulated to meet specific calorie and nutritional targets.

- Variety of Foods: Jenny Craig meals include a range of options such as pasta dishes, pizzas, burgers, soups, salads, and desserts.

- Fresh Additions: Participants are encouraged to supplement Jenny Craig meals with fresh fruits, vegetables, and dairy for added nutrition and variety.

- Snacks: Jenny Craig provides snacks such as bars, shakes, and cookies to help curb hunger between meals.

- Flexibility: Jenny Craig offers flexibility with "Your List," allowing participants to incorporate their favorite foods into their meal plans in moderation.

Instructions/How to Prepare:

1. Enroll in the Jenny Craig program and choose a meal plan based on individual weight loss goals, dietary preferences, and lifestyle.

2. Receive pre-packaged meals and snacks delivered to your home or pick them up at a Jenny Craig center, following the meal plan and eating schedule provided.

3. Enjoy Jenny Craig meals and snacks as directed, incorporating fresh fruits, vegetables, and dairy as recommended for added nutrition and variety.

4. Supplement Jenny Craig meals with water or other non-caloric beverages to stay hydrated throughout the day.

5. Schedule one-on-one coaching sessions with a Jenny Craig consultant to receive personalized support, guidance, and encouragement throughout the weight loss journey.

6. Utilize support tools such as online resources, meal planners, and the Jenny Craig app to track progress, access meal plans, and stay motivated.

7. Incorporate physical activity into daily routines to complement Jenny Craig's weight loss program and promote overall health and well-being.

8. Practice portion control and mindful eating by savoring each bite and paying attention to hunger and fullness cues.

9. Monitor weight loss progress and adjust meal plans as needed to achieve and maintain desired results.

10. Continue following Jenny Craig's maintenance plan and lifestyle recommendations to sustain weight loss and promote long-term success.

SlimFast Diet:

Definition:

The SlimFast Diet is a popular commercial weight loss program that revolves around meal replacement shakes, bars, and snacks. It offers a structured plan designed to help individuals lose weight by replacing two meals a day with SlimFast products and enjoying one sensible meal and three low-calorie snacks. The program provides portion-controlled, calorie-controlled meals and encourages participants to follow a balanced diet, incorporating fruits, vegetables, lean proteins, and whole grains alongside SlimFast products. Additionally, SlimFast offers support tools, online resources, and a community for motivation and accountability.

Ingredients:

- SlimFast Shakes: Meal replacement shakes available in various flavors, formulated to provide essential nutrients and promote satiety.

- SlimFast Bars: Meal replacement bars available in different flavors, offering a convenient and portable option for on-the-go nutrition.

- SlimFast Snacks: Low-calorie snacks such as snack bars, chips, and crisps designed to satisfy hunger between meals.

Instructions/How to Prepare:

1. Choose a SlimFast plan based on individual weight loss goals, dietary preferences, and lifestyle.

2. Replace two meals a day with SlimFast shakes or bars, enjoying one sensible meal and three low-calorie snacks.

3. Follow the SlimFast meal plan and eating schedule, incorporating fruits, vegetables, lean proteins, and whole grains into sensible meals and snacks.

4. Drink plenty of water throughout the day to stay hydrated and promote overall health and well-being.

5. Utilize support tools such as online resources, meal planners, and the SlimFast app to track progress, access meal plans, and stay motivated.

6. Incorporate physical activity into daily routines to complement the SlimFast weight loss program and promote overall fitness and well-being.

7. Practice portion control and mindful eating by paying attention to hunger and fullness cues and savoring each bite.

8. Monitor weight loss progress and adjust meal plans as needed to achieve and maintain desired results.

9. Continue following the SlimFast maintenance plan and lifestyle recommendations to sustain weight loss and promote long-term success.

10. Seek support from the SlimFast community, including counselors, fellow participants, and online forums, for motivation, encouragement, and accountability throughout the weight loss journey.

Volumetrics Diet:

Definition:

The Volumetrics Diet, developed by Barbara Rolls, PhD, emphasizes eating high-volume, low-calorie foods to promote satiety and weight loss. It focuses on consuming foods that are low in energy density (calories per gram) but high in volume, such as fruits, vegetables, whole grains, and lean proteins. By emphasizing foods with high water content, fiber, and nutrients, the Volumetrics Diet aims to help individuals feel full and satisfied while consuming fewer calories. The diet offers flexibility and variety, allowing participants to enjoy a wide range of foods while still achieving weight loss goals.

Ingredients:

- Fruits: Berries, apples, oranges, bananas, mangoes, melons, etc.

- Vegetables: Leafy greens, broccoli, cauliflower, bell peppers, carrots, onions, etc.

- Whole Grains: Brown rice, quinoa, oats, barley, whole wheat bread, whole grain pasta.

- Lean Proteins: Chicken, turkey, fish, seafood, tofu, tempeh, lean cuts of beef or pork.

- Healthy Fats: Avocado, nuts, seeds, olive oil.

- Low-Calorie Foods: Soups, salads, broth-based dishes, fruits, vegetables, and foods with high water content and low energy density.

Instructions/How to Prepare:

1. Familiarize yourself with the concept of energy density and how it influences food choices and portion sizes.

2. Focus on consuming foods that are low in energy density, such as fruits, vegetables, whole grains, and lean proteins, as the foundation of meals and snacks.

3. Prioritize water-rich foods like soups, salads, and broth-based dishes to increase meal volume without adding extra calories.

4. Incorporate fiber-rich foods such as fruits, vegetables, whole grains, and legumes to promote satiety and support digestive health.

5. Use portion control techniques such as measuring food portions, using smaller plates, and being mindful of serving sizes to manage calorie intake.

6. Be strategic with meal planning and food choices, opting for nutrient-dense foods that provide essential vitamins, minerals, and antioxidants.

7. Include a variety of flavors, textures, and colors in meals to enhance satisfaction and enjoyment.

8. Practice mindful eating by paying attention to hunger and fullness cues, eating slowly, and savoring each bite.

9. Stay hydrated by drinking plenty of water throughout the day, as thirst can sometimes be mistaken for hunger.

10. Monitor weight loss progress and adjust meal plans as needed to achieve and maintain desired results while incorporating lifelong habits for long-term health and well-being.

SparkPeople Diet:

Definition:

The SparkPeople Diet is an online weight loss and wellness program that offers tools, resources, and support for individuals looking to achieve their health and fitness goals. The program provides personalized meal plans, workout routines, tracking tools, and a supportive community to help participants make sustainable lifestyle changes. The SparkPeople Diet focuses on a balanced approach to nutrition, exercise, and behavior change, emphasizing portion control, mindful eating, and regular physical activity. It encourages participants to set realistic goals, track progress, and celebrate successes along the way.

Ingredients:

- Balanced Meals: SparkPeople provides personalized meal plans tailored to individual dietary preferences, calorie needs, and weight loss goals.

- Nutrient-Dense Foods: Participants are encouraged to incorporate a variety of fruits, vegetables, whole grains, lean proteins, and healthy fats into their meals and snacks.

- Portion Control: SparkPeople emphasizes portion control techniques such as measuring food portions, using smaller plates, and being mindful of serving sizes to manage calorie intake.

- Exercise Routines: SparkPeople offers workout routines and fitness videos for participants to incorporate regular physical activity into their daily routines.

- Tracking Tools: SparkPeople provides tracking tools for food intake, exercise, weight loss progress, and other health metrics to help participants stay accountable and monitor their success.

- Supportive Community: SparkPeople offers a supportive online community where participants can connect with others, share experiences, and receive encouragement and motivation.

Instructions/How to Prepare:

1. Sign up for the SparkPeople program and create a personalized profile, including information about dietary preferences, weight loss goals, and activity level.

2. Receive personalized meal plans, workout routines, and tracking tools based on individual needs and goals.

3. Follow the SparkPeople meal plan, incorporating a variety of nutrient-dense foods such as fruits, vegetables, whole grains, lean proteins, and healthy fats into meals and snacks.

4. Practice portion control by measuring food portions, using smaller plates, and being mindful of serving sizes to manage calorie intake.

5. Incorporate regular physical activity into daily routines, following SparkPeople workout routines and fitness videos or engaging in other forms of exercise that are enjoyable and sustainable.

6. Use SparkPeople tracking tools to monitor food intake, exercise, weight loss progress, and other health metrics, staying accountable and motivated along the way.

7. Engage with the SparkPeople community, connecting with others, sharing experiences, and receiving encouragement and support throughout the weight loss journey.

8. Be patient and consistent, recognizing that weight loss and lifestyle changes take time and effort, and celebrating successes along the way.

9. Adjust meal plans, workout routines, and goals as needed based on progress and feedback, staying flexible and adaptable to individual needs and preferences.

10. Embrace a lifelong commitment to health and wellness, incorporating healthy habits into daily life and continuing to strive for improvement and success.

The Fast Diet (5:2 Diet):

Definition:

The Fast Diet, also known as the 5:2 Diet, is a popular intermittent fasting approach that involves alternating between regular eating days and fasting days. On fasting days, individuals restrict calorie intake to a quarter of their usual daily intake, typically around 500-600 calories for women and 600-800 calories for men. On non-fasting days, individuals eat normally without calorie restriction. The Fast Diet is believed to promote weight loss, improve metabolic health, and provide other potential health benefits by inducing a state of mild calorie restriction and metabolic adaptation.

Ingredients:

- Regular Eating Days: On non-fasting days, individuals can eat a balanced diet that includes a variety of foods such as fruits, vegetables, whole grains, lean proteins, and healthy fats.

- Fasting Days: On fasting days, individuals consume a limited number of calories, typically from low-calorie foods such as vegetables, fruits, lean proteins, and small amounts of grains and fats.

- Fluids: Adequate hydration is important on fasting days, so drinking water, herbal tea, and other non-caloric beverages is encouraged.

Instructions/How to Prepare:

1. Determine fasting days and non-fasting days based on personal preferences, lifestyle, and schedule.

2. Plan meals and snacks for non-fasting days that provide balanced nutrition and meet individual dietary preferences and calorie needs.

3. On fasting days, consume a limited number of calories, typically around 500-600 calories for women and 600-800 calories for men, spread throughout the day.

4. Choose low-calorie foods that provide satiety and essential nutrients, such as vegetables, fruits, lean proteins, and small amounts of grains and fats.

5. Practice portion control and mindful eating on both fasting and non-fasting days to manage calorie intake and support overall health and well-being.

6. Stay hydrated by drinking plenty of water throughout the day, especially on fasting days when calorie intake is restricted.

7. Consider experimenting with different fasting schedules, such as alternate-day fasting or modified fasting, to find what works best for individual preferences and goals.

8. Be patient and flexible, recognizing that intermittent fasting may take time to adapt to and may not be suitable for everyone.

9. Monitor hunger, energy levels, and overall well-being throughout the fasting period, adjusting dietary choices and fasting schedules as needed.

10. Consult with a healthcare professional or registered dietitian before starting the Fast Diet, especially if you have underlying health conditions or concerns about fasting.

The Warrior Diet:

Definition:

The Warrior Diet is an intermittent fasting approach that involves extended periods of fasting followed by short eating windows.

Inspired by ancient warrior cultures, this diet encourages individuals to fast for approximately 20 hours each day and consume one large meal during a 4-hour "overeating" window in the evening. During the fasting period, individuals are encouraged to consume small amounts of raw fruits, vegetables, and non-caloric beverages to support hydration and provide minimal energy. The Warrior Diet is believed to promote fat loss, improve metabolic health, and increase mental clarity and focus by aligning eating patterns with natural circadian rhythms.

Ingredients:

- Fasting Period: During the fasting period, individuals consume small amounts of raw fruits, vegetables, and non-caloric beverages such as water, herbal tea, or black coffee.

- Overeating Window: During the overeating window, individuals consume one large meal that includes a variety of nutrient-dense foods such as lean proteins, whole grains, fruits, vegetables, healthy fats, and dairy or dairy alternatives.

Instructions/How to Prepare:

1. Determine fasting and eating windows based on personal preferences, lifestyle, and schedule.

2. Start the day with hydration by drinking water, herbal tea, or black coffee during the fasting period to support overall health and well-being.

3. Consume small amounts of raw fruits and vegetables throughout the fasting period to help manage hunger and provide essential nutrients.

4. Break the fast with a large, nutrient-dense meal during the overeating window, incorporating a variety of foods such as lean proteins, whole grains, fruits, vegetables, healthy fats, and dairy or dairy alternatives.

5. Practice mindful eating during the overeating window, focusing on hunger and fullness cues and savoring each bite of food.

6. Stay hydrated throughout the day by drinking plenty of water and other non-caloric beverages to support hydration and overall health.

7. Experiment with different meal compositions and timing strategies to find what works best for individual preferences and goals.

8. Listen to your body and adjust eating patterns as needed based on hunger, energy levels, and overall well-being.

9. Be patient and flexible, recognizing that intermittent fasting may take time to adapt to and may not be suitable for everyone.

10.   Consult with a healthcare professional or registered dietitian before starting the Warrior Diet, especially if you have underlying health conditions or concerns about fasting.

The Blood Sugar Solution Diet:

Definition:

The Blood Sugar Solution Diet, developed by Dr. Mark Hyman, is a comprehensive approach to managing blood sugar levels and promoting overall health and well-being. It focuses on reducing inflammation, balancing blood sugar, and optimizing metabolism through dietary changes, lifestyle modifications, and targeted supplementation. The diet emphasizes whole, nutrient-dense foods that support stable blood sugar levels, such as non-starchy vegetables, lean proteins, healthy fats, and low-glycemic carbohydrates. It also encourages individuals to eliminate processed foods, refined sugars, artificial additives, and other inflammatory substances from their diet to reduce insulin resistance and improve metabolic function.

Ingredients:

- Whole Foods: Non-starchy vegetables, leafy greens, lean proteins, nuts, seeds, legumes, whole grains, healthy fats, and low-glycemic fruits are emphasized on The Blood Sugar Solution Diet.

- Nutrient-Dense Foods: Foods rich in essential nutrients, vitamins, minerals, and antioxidants are prioritized to support overall health and well-being.

- Elimination of Processed Foods: Processed foods, refined sugars, artificial additives, trans fats, and other inflammatory substances are eliminated or minimized to reduce inflammation and support metabolic health.

- Hydration: Adequate hydration is important on The Blood Sugar Solution Diet, so drinking water, herbal tea, and other non-caloric beverages is encouraged.

Instructions/How to Prepare:

1. Familiarize yourself with the principles of The Blood Sugar Solution Diet, including recommendations for food choices, portion sizes, meal timing, and lifestyle habits.

2. Stock your kitchen with whole, nutrient-dense foods such as non-starchy vegetables, leafy greens, lean proteins, nuts, seeds, legumes, whole grains, healthy fats, and low-glycemic fruits.

3. Plan meals and snacks that prioritize whole foods and balance macronutrients to support stable blood sugar levels and optimize metabolism.

4. Focus on eating a variety of colors, flavors, and textures in meals to ensure a diverse intake of nutrients and promote satiety and enjoyment.

5. Minimize or eliminate processed foods, refined sugars, artificial additives, trans fats, and other inflammatory substances from your diet to reduce inflammation and support metabolic health.

6. Pay attention to portion sizes and practice mindful eating by listening to hunger and fullness cues, eating slowly, and savoring each bite.

7. Stay hydrated by drinking plenty of water throughout the day to support overall health and well-being.

8. Incorporate regular physical activity into your daily routine to enhance metabolic function, support weight management, and promote overall fitness and well-being.

9. Monitor blood sugar levels regularly, especially for individuals with diabetes or insulin resistance, and adjust dietary choices as needed to achieve and maintain optimal blood sugar control.

10. Consult with a healthcare professional or registered dietitian before starting The Blood Sugar Solution Diet, especially if you have underlying health conditions or concerns about dietary changes.

The Insulin-Resistance Diet:

Definition:

The Insulin-Resistance Diet is a dietary approach aimed at managing insulin resistance, a condition in which cells become less responsive to the effects of insulin, leading to elevated blood sugar levels. This diet focuses on regulating blood sugar levels, improving insulin sensitivity, and promoting overall health and well-being. It emphasizes whole, nutrient-dense foods that have a minimal impact on blood sugar levels, such as non-starchy vegetables, lean proteins, healthy fats, and high-fiber carbohydrates. The Insulin-Resistance Diet also encourages regular physical activity, stress management, and lifestyle modifications to support metabolic health.

Ingredients:

- Whole Foods: Non-starchy vegetables, leafy greens, lean proteins, nuts, seeds, legumes, whole grains, healthy fats, and low-glycemic fruits are emphasized on The Insulin-Resistance Diet.

- High-Fiber Carbohydrates: Carbohydrates with a high fiber content, such as whole grains, legumes, fruits, and vegetables, are preferred to support stable blood sugar levels and promote satiety.

- Lean Proteins: Lean sources of protein, including poultry, fish, tofu, tempeh, legumes, and low-fat dairy products, are prioritized to support muscle health and metabolic function.

- Healthy Fats: Monounsaturated and polyunsaturated fats from sources such as avocados, nuts, seeds, olive oil, and fatty fish are encouraged to provide essential nutrients and support cardiovascular health.

- Low-Glycemic Foods: Foods with a low glycemic index, which have a minimal impact on blood sugar levels, are favored on The Insulin-Resistance Diet to help regulate insulin levels and prevent spikes and crashes in blood sugar.

Instructions/How to Prepare:

1. Educate yourself about insulin resistance and how dietary and lifestyle factors can influence blood sugar levels and insulin sensitivity.

2. Stock your kitchen with whole, nutrient-dense foods such as non-starchy vegetables, leafy greens, lean proteins, nuts, seeds, legumes, whole grains, healthy fats, and low-glycemic fruits.

3. Plan meals and snacks that prioritize whole foods and balance macronutrients to support stable blood sugar levels and improve insulin sensitivity.

4. Focus on eating a variety of colors, flavors, and textures in meals to ensure a diverse intake of nutrients and promote satiety and enjoyment.

5. Choose high-fiber carbohydrates such as whole grains, legumes, fruits, and vegetables to slow the absorption of sugar into the bloodstream and prevent spikes in blood sugar levels.

6. Incorporate lean sources of protein into meals and snacks to support muscle health, promote satiety, and stabilize blood sugar levels.

7. Include healthy fats from sources such as avocados, nuts, seeds, olive oil, and fatty fish to provide essential nutrients and support cardiovascular health.

8. Minimize or eliminate processed foods, refined sugars, artificial additives, trans fats, and other inflammatory substances from your diet to reduce inflammation and improve metabolic health.

9. Pay attention to portion sizes and practice mindful eating by listening to hunger and fullness cues, eating slowly, and savoring each bite.

10. Stay hydrated by drinking plenty of water throughout the day to support overall health and well-being.

The Sugar Busters Diet:

Definition:

The Sugar Busters Diet is a low-glycemic approach to eating that aims to control blood sugar levels and promote weight loss by minimizing the consumption of high-glycemic carbohydrates and sugars. It emphasizes whole, nutrient-dense foods that have a minimal impact on blood sugar levels, such as non-starchy vegetables, lean proteins, healthy fats, and low-glycemic carbohydrates. The Sugar Busters Diet also encourages portion control, regular physical activity, and lifestyle modifications to support metabolic health and overall well-being.

Ingredients:

- Whole Foods: Non-starchy vegetables, leafy greens, lean proteins, nuts, seeds, legumes, whole grains, healthy fats, and low-glycemic fruits are emphasized on The Sugar Busters Diet.

- Low-Glycemic Carbohydrates: Carbohydrates with a low glycemic index, such as whole grains, legumes, fruits, and vegetables, are preferred to help regulate blood sugar levels and prevent spikes and crashes in blood sugar.

- Lean Proteins: Lean sources of protein, including poultry, fish, tofu, tempeh, legumes, and low-fat dairy products, are prioritized to support muscle health and metabolic function.

- Healthy Fats: Monounsaturated and polyunsaturated fats from sources such as avocados, nuts, seeds, olive oil, and fatty fish are encouraged to provide essential nutrients and support cardiovascular health.

Instructions/How to Prepare:

1. Familiarize yourself with the principles of The Sugar Busters Diet, including recommendations for food choices, portion sizes, meal timing, and lifestyle habits.

2. Stock your kitchen with whole, nutrient-dense foods such as non-starchy vegetables, leafy greens, lean proteins, nuts, seeds, legumes, whole grains, healthy fats, and low-glycemic fruits.

3. Plan meals and snacks that prioritize whole foods and balance macronutrients to support stable blood sugar levels and improve insulin sensitivity.

4. Focus on eating a variety of colors, flavors, and textures in meals to ensure a diverse intake of nutrients and promote satiety and enjoyment.

5. Choose low-glycemic carbohydrates such as whole grains, legumes, fruits, and vegetables to help regulate blood sugar levels and prevent spikes and crashes in blood sugar.

6. Incorporate lean sources of protein into meals and snacks to support muscle health, promote satiety, and stabilize blood sugar levels.

7. Include healthy fats from sources such as avocados, nuts, seeds, olive oil, and fatty fish to provide essential nutrients and support cardiovascular health.

8. Practice portion control by measuring food portions, using smaller plates, and being mindful of serving sizes to manage calorie intake and support weight loss.

9. Stay hydrated by drinking plenty of water throughout the day to support overall health and well-being.

10. Incorporate regular physical activity into your daily routine to enhance metabolic function, support weight management, and promote overall fitness and well-being.

CHAPTER 11

DIET FOR DIABETES

Mediterranean Diet:

Definition:

The Mediterranean diet is inspired by the traditional dietary patterns of countries bordering the Mediterranean Sea. It emphasizes whole, minimally processed foods such as fruits, vegetables, whole grains, nuts, seeds, legumes, fish, and olive oil. It limits red meat and sweets, while encouraging moderate consumption of dairy products, poultry, and eggs.

Ingredients:

- Fruits: Berries, apples, oranges, grapes, etc.

- Vegetables: Spinach, tomatoes, peppers, onions, etc.

- Whole Grains: Whole wheat bread, brown rice, quinoa, oats, etc.

- Nuts and Seeds: Almonds, walnuts, flaxseeds, chia seeds, etc.

- Legumes: Chickpeas, lentils, beans, etc.

- Fish and Seafood: Salmon, tuna, shrimp, etc.

- Olive Oil: Extra virgin olive oil for cooking and dressing.

- Herbs and Spices: Basil, oregano, garlic, cumin, etc.

Instructions/How to Prepare:

1. Base meals around plant-based foods like fruits, vegetables, whole grains, and legumes.

2. Use olive oil as the primary source of fat for cooking and dressing salads.

3. Incorporate fish and seafood into your diet regularly, aiming for at least two servings per week.

4. Enjoy moderate amounts of poultry, eggs, and dairy products, such as yogurt and cheese.

5. Limit red meat consumption to a few times per month.

6. Snack on nuts and seeds for a healthy source of fats and protein.

7. Flavor meals with herbs and spices instead of salt.

8. Drink plenty of water and enjoy a moderate amount of red wine if desired (optional).

DASH Diet (Dietary Approaches to Stop Hypertension):

Definition:

The DASH diet is specifically designed to help lower blood pressure and reduce the risk of hypertension. It emphasizes fruits, vegetables, whole grains, and lean proteins while limiting sodium, saturated fats, and sweets.

Ingredients:

- Fruits: Berries, bananas, apples, oranges, etc.
- Vegetables: Leafy greens, carrots, broccoli, bell peppers, etc.
- Whole Grains: Brown rice, whole wheat bread, quinoa, oats, barley, etc.
- Lean Proteins: Chicken breast, turkey, fish, tofu, beans, lentils, etc.
- Dairy: Low-fat or fat-free milk, yogurt, cheese, etc.
- Nuts and Seeds: Almonds, pistachios, sunflower seeds, etc.
- Healthy Fats: Olive oil, avocado, nuts, seeds, etc.

Instructions/How to Prepare:

1. Focus on incorporating plenty of fruits and vegetables into your meals and snacks.
2. Choose whole grains over refined grains whenever possible.
3. Opt for lean proteins such as poultry, fish, tofu, and legumes.
4. Limit high-fat dairy products and opt for low-fat or fat-free options.
5. Include nuts and seeds as snacks or in salads for added nutrients and healthy fats.

6. Use herbs, spices, and citrus juices to flavor foods instead of salt.

7. Avoid processed and high-sodium foods like canned soups, packaged snacks, and fast food.

8. Cook meals at home whenever possible to have better control over ingredients and portion sizes.

9. Aim to limit sweets and sugary beverages, opting for natural sweeteners like fruit when craving something sweet.

10. Stay hydrated by drinking plenty of water throughout the day.

Low-Carb Diet:

Definition:

A low-carb diet involves reducing carbohydrate intake while increasing the consumption of protein and healthy fats. This diet aims to control insulin levels, promote weight loss, and improve overall health by limiting foods high in carbohydrates such as bread, pasta, rice, and sugary snacks.

Ingredients:

- Protein Sources: Meat, poultry, fish, tofu, tempeh, eggs.

- Non-Starchy Vegetables: Leafy greens, broccoli, cauliflower, zucchini, bell peppers.

- Healthy Fats: Avocado, nuts, seeds, olive oil, coconut oil.

- Dairy: Cheese, Greek yogurt, cottage cheese (in moderation).

- Low-Carb Fruits: Berries, avocados, tomatoes, lemons, limes.

- Herbs and Spices: Basil, oregano, garlic, turmeric, cumin.

- Sweeteners (optional): Stevia, erythritol, monk fruit.

Instructions/How to Prepare:

1. Focus on whole, unprocessed foods.

2. Limit carbohydrate intake to around 20-50 grams per day, depending on individual needs and goals.

3. Include protein-rich foods in each meal to promote satiety and muscle maintenance.

4. Fill up on non-starchy vegetables to increase fiber intake and provide essential vitamins and minerals.

5. Incorporate healthy fats into your diet for energy and to keep you feeling full.

6. Be mindful of hidden carbs in sauces, condiments, and processed foods.

7. Drink plenty of water to stay hydrated and support overall health.

8. Experiment with low-carb recipes and meal prep to make adhering to the diet easier and more enjoyable.

Ketogenic Diet (Keto Diet):

Definition:

The ketogenic diet is a very low-carb, high-fat diet that forces the body to enter a state of ketosis, where it primarily burns fat for fuel instead of carbohydrates. This diet has been used for decades to treat epilepsy and has gained popularity for weight loss and improving metabolic health.

Ingredients:

- Healthy Fats: Avocado, coconut oil, olive oil, butter, ghee, fatty fish.

- Protein Sources: Meat, poultry, fish, eggs, tofu, tempeh.

- Non-Starchy Vegetables: Leafy greens, broccoli, cauliflower, zucchini, asparagus.

- Full-Fat Dairy: Cheese, heavy cream, Greek yogurt (in moderation).

- Nuts and Seeds: Macadamia nuts, almonds, chia seeds, flaxseeds.

- Low-Carb Fruits: Berries (in moderation), avocado.

- Herbs and Spices: Turmeric, ginger, cinnamon, garlic, thyme.

- Sweeteners (in moderation): Stevia, erythritol, monk fruit.

Instructions/How to Prepare:

1. Keep carbohydrate intake extremely low, typically below 20-50 grams per day to induce and maintain ketosis.

2. Consume moderate amounts of protein, as excessive protein intake can potentially hinder ketosis.

3. Base meals around healthy fats, such as avocados, olive oil, and fatty fish.

4. Incorporate non-starchy vegetables to provide essential nutrients and fiber while keeping carbohydrate intake low.

5. Be mindful of hidden carbs in foods and beverages, including sauces, dressings, and flavored beverages.

6. Stay hydrated by drinking plenty of water, as dehydration can occur more easily on a ketogenic diet.

7. Monitor ketone levels using urine strips, blood tests, or breath meters if desired, to ensure you are in ketosis.

8. Experiment with keto-friendly recipes and meal planning to maintain variety and enjoyment while following the diet.

Plant-Based Diet:

Definition:

A plant-based diet primarily consists of foods derived from plants, such as fruits, vegetables, grains, nuts, seeds, and legumes. It emphasizes whole, minimally processed foods while minimizing or eliminating animal products. The focus is on incorporating a variety of plant foods to promote health and well-being.

Ingredients:

- Fruits: Berries, apples, oranges, bananas, etc.

- Vegetables: Leafy greens, broccoli, carrots, bell peppers, etc.

- Whole Grains: Brown rice, quinoa, oats, barley, whole wheat bread, etc.

- Legumes: Chickpeas, lentils, black beans, kidney beans, etc.

- Nuts and Seeds: Almonds, walnuts, chia seeds, flaxseeds, pumpkin seeds, etc.

- Plant-Based Proteins: Tofu, tempeh, seitan, edamame, plant-based protein powders, etc.

- Healthy Fats: Avocado, olive oil, coconut oil, nuts, seeds, etc.

Instructions/How to Prepare:

1. Base meals around a variety of whole plant foods, including fruits, vegetables, whole grains, legumes, nuts, and seeds.

2. Incorporate a rainbow of colorful fruits and vegetables to ensure a diverse array of nutrients.

3. Include plant-based proteins such as tofu, tempeh, and legumes in meals to meet protein needs.

4. Choose whole grains over refined grains for added fiber and nutrients.

5. Experiment with different cooking methods, such as steaming, roasting, sautéing, and grilling, to enhance flavor and texture.

6. Use herbs, spices, and condiments to add flavor to dishes without relying on animal products.

7. Be mindful of nutrient needs, particularly vitamin B12, vitamin D, omega-3 fatty acids, iron, calcium, and zinc, and consider supplementation if necessary.

8. Stay hydrated by drinking plenty of water throughout the day.

9. Plan balanced meals and snacks to ensure adequate intake of essential nutrients.

10. Enjoy plant-based alternatives to dairy and meat products, such as plant-based milk, cheese, yogurt, and meat substitutes, if desired.

Vegan Diet:

Definition:

A vegan diet excludes all animal products, including meat, poultry, fish, dairy, eggs, and honey. It is based entirely on plant foods and emphasizes cruelty-free living and environmental sustainability.

Ingredients:

- Fruits: Berries, apples, oranges, mangoes, etc.

- Vegetables: Spinach, kale, tomatoes, onions, mushrooms, etc.

- Whole Grains: Quinoa, brown rice, barley, whole wheat pasta, etc.

- Legumes: Chickpeas, black beans, lentils, kidney beans, etc.

- Nuts and Seeds: Almonds, cashews, sunflower seeds, chia seeds, etc.

- Plant-Based Proteins: Tofu, tempeh, seitan, soy-based meat substitutes, etc.

- Healthy Fats: Avocado, olive oil, coconut oil, nuts, seeds, etc.

- Plant-Based Dairy Alternatives: Almond milk, coconut milk, soy milk, vegan cheese, vegan yogurt, etc.

Instructions/How to Prepare:

1. Build meals around plant foods, including fruits, vegetables, whole grains, legumes, nuts, and seeds.

2. Ensure adequate protein intake by including sources such as tofu, tempeh, legumes, and plant-based meat substitutes.

3. Use plant-based milk, cheese, and yogurt alternatives in place of dairy products.

4. Experiment with vegan cooking techniques and recipes to discover new flavors and textures.

5. Pay attention to nutrient needs, especially vitamin B12, vitamin D, omega-3 fatty acids, iron, calcium, and zinc, and consider supplementation if necessary.

6. Read labels carefully to avoid hidden animal ingredients in processed foods and beverages.

7. Be mindful of cross-contamination when preparing and consuming food to prevent unintentional consumption of animal products.

8. Explore vegan-friendly restaurants and eateries or plan ahead when dining out to ensure vegan options are available.

9. Connect with vegan communities and resources for support, recipe ideas, and lifestyle tips.

10.   Embrace the ethical and environmental principles of veganism beyond diet by choosing cruelty-free and

sustainable products in other areas of life, such as clothing, cosmetics, and household items.

Vegetarian Diet:

Definition:

A vegetarian diet excludes meat, poultry, and seafood, but includes plant-based foods such as fruits, vegetables, grains, nuts, seeds, and dairy products. There are different variations of vegetarianism, including lacto-vegetarian (includes dairy but not eggs), ovo-vegetarian (includes eggs but not dairy), and lacto-ovo-vegetarian (includes both dairy and eggs).

Ingredients:

- Fruits: Berries, apples, oranges, bananas, etc.

- Vegetables: Leafy greens, broccoli, carrots, bell peppers, etc.

- Whole Grains: Brown rice, quinoa, oats, barley, whole wheat bread, etc.

- Legumes: Chickpeas, lentils, black beans, kidney beans, etc.

- Nuts and Seeds: Almonds, walnuts, chia seeds, flaxseeds, pumpkin seeds, etc.

- Dairy: Milk, yogurt, cheese, butter, etc. (depending on the type of vegetarianism)

- Plant-Based Proteins: Tofu, tempeh, seitan, edamame, etc.

- Healthy Fats: Avocado, olive oil, coconut oil, nuts, seeds, etc.

Instructions/How to Prepare:

1. Base meals around a variety of plant foods, including fruits, vegetables, whole grains, legumes, nuts, and seeds.

2. Incorporate plant-based proteins such as tofu, tempeh, legumes, nuts, and seeds into meals to meet protein needs.

3. Choose whole grains over refined grains for added fiber and nutrients.

4. Experiment with different cooking methods, such as steaming, roasting, sautéing, and grilling, to enhance flavor and texture.

5. Use herbs, spices, and condiments to add flavor to dishes without relying on meat.

6. Be mindful of nutrient needs, especially vitamin B12, vitamin D, omega-3 fatty acids, iron, calcium, and zinc, and consider supplementation if necessary.

7. Stay hydrated by drinking plenty of water throughout the day.

8. Plan balanced meals and snacks to ensure adequate intake of essential nutrients.

9. Explore vegetarian cooking techniques and recipes to discover new flavors and textures.

10. Connect with vegetarian communities and resources for support, recipe ideas, and lifestyle tips.

Glycemic Load Diet:

Definition:

The Glycemic Load Diet focuses on managing blood sugar levels by selecting foods based on their glycemic load, which takes into account both the quality and quantity of carbohydrates in a serving of food. The diet aims to minimize blood sugar spikes and promote stable energy levels by emphasizing foods with a low glycemic load, such as fruits, vegetables, whole grains, lean proteins, and healthy fats. It encourages portion control, balanced meals, and mindful eating to support overall health and well-being.

Ingredients:

- Low-Glycemic Foods: Fruits, vegetables, whole grains, legumes, nuts, seeds, lean proteins, and healthy fats.

- High-Fiber Foods: Foods high in fiber such as fruits, vegetables, whole grains, legumes, nuts, and seeds can help slow the absorption of carbohydrates and promote satiety.

- Healthy Fats: Avocado, nuts, seeds, olive oil, fatty fish (salmon, mackerel, sardines) provide essential nutrients and help balance blood sugar levels.

- Lean Proteins: Chicken, turkey, fish, seafood, tofu, tempeh, lean cuts of beef or pork provide satiety and support muscle health.

- Portion-Controlled Carbohydrates: Portion control is emphasized to manage carbohydrate intake and prevent blood sugar spikes.

Instructions/How to Prepare:

1. Understand the concept of glycemic load and how it influences blood sugar levels and overall health.

2. Choose foods with a low glycemic load, such as fruits, vegetables, whole grains, legumes, nuts, seeds, lean proteins, and healthy fats, as the foundation of meals and snacks.

3. Emphasize high-fiber foods to promote satiety, stabilize blood sugar levels, and support digestive health.

4. Incorporate healthy fats into meals and snacks to balance blood sugar levels and promote feelings of fullness and satisfaction.

5. Include lean proteins in meals to provide essential nutrients, promote muscle health, and support satiety.

6. Practice portion control by measuring food portions, using smaller plates, and being mindful of serving sizes to manage carbohydrate intake.

7. Be mindful of meal timing and spacing to prevent blood sugar spikes and maintain stable energy levels throughout the day.

8. Monitor blood sugar levels regularly, especially for individuals with diabetes or insulin resistance, and adjust dietary choices as needed to achieve and maintain optimal blood sugar control.

9. Stay hydrated by drinking plenty of water throughout the day to support overall health and well-being.

10. Seek guidance from a healthcare professional or registered dietitian experienced in glycemic load and blood sugar management for personalized recommendations and support.

Low-Protein Diet:

Definition:

A low-protein diet is a dietary approach that restricts the intake of protein-rich foods, often for medical reasons. It may be prescribed for individuals with certain kidney conditions, liver disease, or metabolic disorders that impair protein metabolism. The diet typically limits high-protein foods such as meat, poultry, fish, eggs, dairy products, and legumes while allowing moderate consumption of low-protein foods such as fruits, vegetables, grains, and fats. The goal of a low-protein diet is to reduce the workload on the kidneys and liver, manage symptoms, and slow the progression of underlying medical conditions.

Ingredients:

- Low-Protein Foods: Fruits, vegetables, grains, fats, and oils are typically allowed in moderate amounts on a low-protein diet.

- Limited Protein Sources: Protein-rich foods such as meat, poultry, fish, eggs, dairy products, and legumes are restricted or limited in portion size.

- Protein-Free Foods: Certain foods may be completely avoided on a low-protein diet, especially those with high protein content.

- Fluids: Adequate hydration is important on a low-protein diet, so drinking water and other low-protein beverages is encouraged.

Instructions/How to Prepare:

1. Consult with a healthcare professional or registered dietitian to determine if a low-protein diet is appropriate for your medical condition and health needs.

2. Receive personalized guidance on the recommended daily intake of protein, as well as specific dietary restrictions and allowances.

3. Identify high-protein foods to limit or avoid, including meat, poultry, fish, eggs, dairy products, and legumes.

4. Plan meals and snacks that emphasize low-protein foods such as fruits, vegetables, grains, and fats while limiting protein-rich ingredients.

5. Use portion control techniques to manage protein intake and ensure compliance with dietary recommendations.

6. Explore alternative protein sources that are lower in protein content, such as tofu, tempeh, seitan, and certain grains and vegetables.

7. Monitor symptoms and adjust dietary choices as needed based on individual tolerance and response to the low-protein diet.

8. Stay hydrated by drinking plenty of water throughout the day, as adequate fluid intake is important for kidney function and overall health.

9. Consider working with a registered dietitian experienced in medical nutrition therapy to develop a customized meal plan and receive ongoing support and guidance.

10.   Regularly follow up with healthcare providers to assess progress, monitor kidney function, and adjust dietary recommendations as needed.

Here's a 31-day meal plan from "The Ultimate Diabetic Cookbook and Meal Plan for the Newly Diagnosed":

Day 1:

- Breakfast: Scrambled eggs with spinach and mushrooms, served with whole grain toast.

- Snack: Greek yogurt with mixed berries.

- Lunch: Grilled chicken salad with mixed greens, cucumber, and cherry tomatoes.

- Snack: Carrot sticks with hummus.

- Dinner: Baked salmon with lemon and dill, served with roasted asparagus and quinoa.

Day 2:

- Breakfast: Overnight oats made with rolled oats, almond milk, chia seeds, and sliced strawberries.

- Snack: Apple slices with almond butter.

- Lunch: Turkey and avocado wrap with whole grain tortilla, lettuce, and tomato.

- Snack: Greek yogurt with a sprinkle of cinnamon.

- Dinner: Beef and vegetable stir-fry with brown rice.

Day 3:

- Breakfast: Whole grain waffles with mixed berries and a dollop of Greek yogurt.

- Snack: Cottage cheese with pineapple chunks.

- Lunch: Lentil soup with a side of whole grain bread.

- Snack: Handful of almonds.

- Dinner: Baked chicken thighs with roasted sweet potatoes and green beans.

Day 4:

- Breakfast: Spinach and feta omelette with a side of sliced oranges.

- Snack: Whole grain crackers with low-fat cheese.

- Lunch: Quinoa salad with black beans, corn, diced bell peppers, and a lime vinaigrette.

- Snack: Celery sticks with peanut butter.

- Dinner: Baked cod with a squeeze of lemon, served with steamed broccoli and wild rice.

Day 5:

- Breakfast: Smoothie made with spinach, banana, almond milk, and protein powder.

- Snack: Cherry tomatoes with mozzarella cheese.

- Lunch: Turkey chili with kidney beans and diced vegetables.

- Snack: Roasted chickpeas.

- Dinner: Stir-fried tofu with mixed vegetables and brown rice.

Day 6:

- Breakfast: Whole grain toast with mashed avocado and poached eggs.

- Snack: Sliced cucumber with hummus.

- Lunch: Grilled shrimp salad with mixed greens, cucumber, and cherry tomatoes.

- Snack: Apple slices with peanut butter.

- Dinner: Vegetable curry with chickpeas, served with quinoa.

Day 7:

- Breakfast: Oatmeal topped with sliced bananas and a sprinkle of cinnamon.

- Snack: Greek yogurt with mixed berries.

- Lunch: Spinach and mushroom whole wheat pizza.

- Snack: Carrot sticks with tzatziki sauce.

- Dinner: Baked turkey meatballs with marinara sauce, served with whole wheat pasta and a side salad.

Day 8:

- Breakfast: Greek yogurt parfait with mixed berries and a sprinkle of granola.

- Snack: Sliced apple with a tablespoon of almond butter.

- Lunch: Turkey and cheese whole wheat wrap with lettuce and tomato.

- Snack: Celery sticks with cream cheese.

- Dinner: Baked salmon with garlic butter sauce, served with roasted Brussels sprouts and quinoa.

Day 9:

- Breakfast: Scrambled eggs with diced bell peppers and onions, served with whole grain toast.

- Snack: Handful of mixed nuts.

- Lunch: Lentil and vegetable stir-fry with brown rice.

- Snack: Cherry tomatoes with mozzarella cheese.

- Dinner: Baked chicken breast with lemon herb seasoning, served with roasted sweet potatoes and green beans.

Day 10:

- Breakfast: Whole grain pancakes with fresh fruit and a drizzle of maple syrup.

- Snack: Carrot sticks with hummus.

- Lunch: Quinoa and black bean stuffed bell peppers, served with a side salad.

- Snack: Greek yogurt with a sprinkle of cinnamon.

- Dinner: Beef and broccoli stir-fry with brown rice.

Day 11:

- Breakfast: Overnight oats with almond milk, chia seeds, and sliced bananas.

- Snack: Apple slices with a tablespoon of peanut butter.

- Lunch: Turkey and avocado salad with mixed greens, cucumber, and cherry tomatoes.

- Snack: Celery sticks with tzatziki sauce.

- Dinner: Baked cod with Mediterranean salsa, served with quinoa and roasted vegetables.

Day 12:

- Breakfast: Spinach and mushroom frittata with a side of mixed berries.

- Snack: Handful of roasted chickpeas.

- Lunch: Lentil soup with a side of whole grain bread.

- Snack: Greek yogurt with mixed berries.

- Dinner: Grilled chicken skewers with bell peppers and onions, served with brown rice.

Day 13:

- Breakfast: Whole grain toast with mashed avocado and sliced tomatoes.

- Snack: Sliced cucumber with hummus.

- Lunch: Turkey chili with kidney beans and diced vegetables.

- Snack: Cherry tomatoes with mozzarella cheese.

- Dinner: Vegetable curry with chickpeas, served with quinoa.

Day 14:

- Breakfast: Oatmeal topped with sliced strawberries and a drizzle of honey.

- Snack: Handful of mixed nuts.

- Lunch: Spinach and feta stuffed chicken breast, served with roasted sweet potatoes.

- Snack: Carrot sticks with cream cheese.

- Dinner: Baked turkey meatballs with marinara sauce, served with whole wheat pasta and a side salad.

Day 15:

- Breakfast: Greek yogurt parfait with mixed berries and a sprinkle of granola.

- Snack: Sliced apple with a tablespoon of almond butter.

- Lunch: Turkey and cheese whole wheat wrap with lettuce and tomato.

- Snack: Celery sticks with hummus.

- Dinner: Baked salmon with garlic butter sauce, served with roasted Brussels sprouts and quinoa.

Day 16:

- Breakfast: Scrambled eggs with diced bell peppers and onions, served with whole grain toast.

- Snack: Handful of mixed nuts.

- Lunch: Lentil and vegetable stir-fry with brown rice.

- Snack: Cherry tomatoes with mozzarella cheese.

- Dinner: Baked chicken breast with lemon herb seasoning, served with roasted sweet potatoes and green beans.

Day 17:

- Breakfast: Whole grain pancakes with fresh fruit and a drizzle of maple syrup.

- Snack: Carrot sticks with hummus.

- Lunch: Quinoa and black bean stuffed bell peppers, served with a side salad.

- Snack: Greek yogurt with a sprinkle of cinnamon.

- Dinner: Beef and broccoli stir-fry with brown rice.

Day 18:

- Breakfast: Overnight oats with almond milk, chia seeds, and sliced bananas.

- Snack: Apple slices with a tablespoon of peanut butter.

- Lunch: Turkey and avocado salad with mixed greens, cucumber, and cherry tomatoes.

- Snack: Celery sticks with tzatziki sauce.

- Dinner: Baked cod with Mediterranean salsa, served with quinoa and roasted vegetables.

Day 19:

- Breakfast: Spinach and mushroom frittata with a side of mixed berries.

- Snack: Handful of roasted chickpeas.

- Lunch: Lentil soup with a side of whole grain bread.

- Snack: Greek yogurt with mixed berries.

- Dinner: Grilled chicken skewers with bell peppers and onions, served with brown rice.

Day 20:

- Breakfast: Whole grain toast with mashed avocado and sliced tomatoes.

- Snack: Sliced cucumber with hummus.

- Lunch: Turkey chili with kidney beans and diced vegetables.

- Snack: Cherry tomatoes with mozzarella cheese.

- Dinner: Vegetable curry with chickpeas, served with quinoa.

Day 21:

- Breakfast: Oatmeal topped with sliced strawberries and a drizzle of honey.

- Snack: Handful of mixed nuts.

- Lunch: Spinach and feta stuffed chicken breast, served with roasted sweet potatoes.

- Snack: Carrot sticks with cream cheese.

- Dinner: Baked turkey meatballs with marinara sauce, served with whole wheat pasta and a side salad.

Day 22:

- Breakfast: Greek yogurt parfait with mixed berries and a sprinkle of granola.

- Snack: Sliced apple with a tablespoon of almond butter.

- Lunch: Turkey and cheese whole wheat wrap with lettuce and tomato.

- Snack: Celery sticks with hummus.

- Dinner: Baked salmon with garlic butter sauce, served with roasted Brussels sprouts and quinoa.

Day 23:

- Breakfast: Scrambled eggs with diced bell peppers and onions, served with whole grain toast.

- Snack: Handful of mixed nuts.

- Lunch: Lentil and vegetable stir-fry with brown rice.

- Snack: Cherry tomatoes with mozzarella cheese.

- Dinner: Baked chicken breast with lemon herb seasoning, served with roasted sweet potatoes and green beans.

Day 24:

- Breakfast: Whole grain pancakes with fresh fruit and a drizzle of maple syrup.

- Snack: Carrot sticks with hummus.

- Lunch: Quinoa and black bean stuffed bell peppers, served with a side salad.

- Snack: Greek yogurt with a sprinkle of cinnamon.

- Dinner: Beef and broccoli stir-fry with brown rice.

Day 25:

- Breakfast: Overnight oats with almond milk, chia seeds, and sliced bananas.

- Snack: Apple slices with a tablespoon of peanut butter.

- Lunch: Turkey and avocado salad with mixed greens, cucumber, and cherry tomatoes.

- Snack: Celery sticks with tzatziki sauce.

- Dinner: Baked cod with Mediterranean salsa, served with quinoa and roasted vegetables.

Day 26:

- Breakfast: Spinach and mushroom frittata with a side of mixed berries.

- Snack: Handful of roasted chickpeas.

- Lunch: Lentil soup with a side of whole grain bread.

- Snack: Greek yogurt with mixed berries.

- Dinner: Grilled chicken skewers with bell peppers and onions, served with brown rice.

Day 27:

- Breakfast: Whole grain toast with mashed avocado and sliced tomatoes.

- Snack: Sliced cucumber with hummus.

- Lunch: Turkey chili with kidney beans and diced vegetables.

- Snack: Cherry tomatoes with mozzarella cheese.

- Dinner: Vegetable curry with chickpeas, served with quinoa.

Day 28:

- Breakfast: Oatmeal topped with sliced strawberries and a drizzle of honey.

- Snack: Handful of mixed nuts.

- Lunch: Spinach and feta stuffed chicken breast, served with roasted sweet potatoes.

- Snack: Carrot sticks with cream cheese.

- Dinner: Baked turkey meatballs with marinara sauce, served with whole wheat pasta and a side salad.

Day 29:

- Breakfast: Greek yogurt parfait with mixed berries and a sprinkle of granola.

- Snack: Sliced apple with a tablespoon of almond butter.

- Lunch: Turkey and cheese whole wheat wrap with lettuce and tomato.

- Snack: Celery sticks with hummus.

- Dinner: Baked salmon with garlic butter sauce, served with roasted Brussels sprouts and quinoa.

Day 30:

- Breakfast: Scrambled eggs with diced bell peppers and onions, served with whole grain toast.

- Snack: Handful of mixed nuts.

- Lunch: Lentil and vegetable stir-fry with brown rice.

- Snack: Cherry tomatoes with mozzarella cheese.

- Dinner: Baked chicken breast with lemon herb seasoning, served with roasted sweet potatoes and green beans.

Day 31:

- Breakfast: Whole grain pancakes with fresh fruit and a drizzle of maple syrup.

- Snack: Carrot sticks with hummus.

- Lunch: Quinoa and black bean stuffed bell peppers, served with a side salad.

- Snack: Greek yogurt with a sprinkle of cinnamon.

- Dinner: Beef and broccoli stir-fry with brown rice.

THE END